Pregnancy and Birth

Dianne Hales

Introduction by C. Everett Koop, M.D., Sc.D.
Former Surgeon General, U.S. Public Health Service

Foreword by Sandra Thurman
Director, Office of National AIDS Policy, The White House

CHELSEA HOUSE PUBLISHERS
Philadelphia

The goal of the 21ST CENTURY HEALTH AND WELLNESS is to provide general information in the ever-changing areas of physiology, psychology, and related medical issues. The titles in this series are not intended to take the place of the professional advice of a physician or other health-care professional.

Chelsea House Publishers
EDITOR IN CHIEF: Stephen Reginald
MANAGING EDITOR: James D. Gallagher
PRODUCTION MANAGER: Pam Loos
ART DIRECTOR: Sara Davis
DIRECTOR OF PHOTOGRAPHY: Judy Hasday
SENIOR PRODUCTION EDITOR: Lee Anne Gelletly
ASSISTANT EDITOR: Anne Hill
PRODUCTION SERVICES: Pre-Press Company, Inc.
COVER DESIGNER/ILLUSTRATOR: Emiliano Begnardi

The Chelsea House World Wide Web site address is http://www.chelseahouse.com

3   5   7   9   8   6   4   2

Library of Congress Cataloging-in-Publication Data

Hales, Dianne R., 1950–

Pregnancy & birth/ by Dianne Hales.
p.   cm — (21st century health and wellness)
Includes bibliographical references and index.
Summary: Examines pregnancy and childbirth, from the beginning of a new life to changes in the family after delivery.
ISBN 0-7910-5527-2 (hc.)
1. Pregnancy—Juvenile literature. 2. Childbirth—Juvenile literature. [1. Pregnancy. 2. Childbirth. 3. Babies.] I. Title: Pregnancy and birth. II. Title. III. 21st century health and wellness.
RG525.5 .H35 1999
618.2—dc21
                                                            99-051569

CONTENTS

- AIDS
- Allergies
- The Circulatory System
- The Digestive System
- The Immune System
- Mononucleosis and Other Infectious Diseases
- Organ Transplants
- Pregnancy & Birth
- The Respiratory System
- Sexually Transmitted Diseases
- Sports Medicine

PREVENTION AND EDUCATION: THE KEYS TO GOOD HEALTH

C. Everett Koop, M.D., Sc.D.
FORMER SURGEON GENERAL,
U.S. Public Health Service

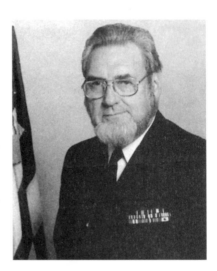

The issue of health education has received particular attention in recent years because of the presence of AIDS in the news. But our response to this particular tragedy points up a number of broader issues that doctors, public health officials, educators, and the public face. In particular, it spotlights the importance of sound health education for citizens of all ages.

Over the past 35 years, this country has been able to achieve dramatic declines in the death rates from heart disease, stroke, accidents, and—for people under the age of 45—cancer. Today, Americans generally eat better and take better care of themselves than ever before. Thus, with the help of modern science and technology, they have a better chance of surviving serious—even catastrophic—illnesses. In 1996, the life expectancy of Americans reached an all-time high of 76.1 years. That's the good news.

The flip side of this advance has special significance for young adults. According to a report issued in 1998 by the U.S. Department of Health and Human Services, levels of wealth and education in the United States are directly correlated with our population's health. The more money Americans make and the more years of schooling they have, the better their health will be. Furthermore, income inequality increased in the U.S. between 1970 and 1996. Basically, the rich got richer—people in high income brackets had greater increases in the amount of money made than did those at low income levels. In addition, the report indicated that children under 18 are more likely to live in poverty than the population as a whole.

Family income rises with each higher level of education for both men and women from every ethnic and racial background. Life expectancy, too, is related to family income. People with lower incomes tend to die at younger ages than people from more affluent homes. What all this means is that health is a factor of wealth and education, both of which need to be improved for all Americans if the promise of life, liberty, and the pursuit of happiness is to include an equal chance for good health.

The health of young people is further threatened by violent death and injury, alcohol and drug abuse, unwanted pregnancies, and sexually transmitted diseases. Adolescents are particularly vulnerable because they are beginning to explore their own sexuality and perhaps to experiment with drugs and alcohol. We need to educate young people to avoid serious dangers to their health. The price of neglect is high.

Even for the population as a whole, health is still far from what it could be. Why? Most death and disease are attributed to four broad elements: inadequacies in the health-care system, behavioral factors or unhealthy lifestyles, environmental hazards, and human biological factors. These categories are also influenced by individual resources. For example, low birth weight and infant mortality are more common among the children of less educated mothers. Likewise, women with more education are more likely to obtain prenatal care during pregnancy. Mothers with fewer than 12 years of education are almost 10 times more likely to smoke during pregnancy—and new studies find excessive aggression later in life as well as other physical ailments among the children of smokers. In short, poor people with less education are more likely to smoke cigarettes, which endangers health and shortens the life span. About a third of the children who begin smoking will eventually have their lives cut short because of this practice.

Similarly, poor children are exposed more often to environmental lead, which causes a wide range of physical and mental problems. Sedentary lifestyles are also more common among teens with lower family income than among wealthier adolescents. Being overweight—a condition associated with physical inactivity as well as excessive caloric intake—is also more common among poor, non-Hispanic, white adolescents. Children from rich families are more likely to have health insurance. Therefore, they are more apt to receive vaccinations and other forms of early preventative medicine and treatment. The bottom line is that kids from lower income groups receive less adequate health care.

To be sure, some diseases are still beyond the control of even the most advanced medical techniques that our richest citizens can afford. Despite yearnings that are as old as the human race itself, there is no "fountain of youth" to prevent aging and death. Still, solutions are available for many of the problems that undermine sound health. In a word, that solution is prevention. Prevention, which includes health promotion and education, can save lives, improve the quality of life, and, in the long run, save money.

In the United States, organized public health activities and preventative medicine have a long history. Important milestones include the improvement of sanitary procedures and the development of pasteurized milk in the late-19th century, and the introduction in the mid-20th century of effective vaccines against polio, measles, German measles, mumps, and other once-rampant diseases. Internationally, organized public health efforts began on a wide-scale basis with the International Sanitary Conference of 1851, to which 12 nations sent representatives. The World Health Organization, founded in 1948, continues these efforts under the aegis of the United Nations, with particular emphasis on combating communicable diseases and the training of health-care workers.

Despite these accomplishments, much remains to be done in the field of prevention. For too long, we have had a medical system that is science and technology-based, and focuses essentially on illness and mortality. It is now patently obvious that both the social and the economic costs of such a system are becoming insupportable.

Implementing prevention and its corollaries, health education and health promotion, is the job of several groups of people. First, the medical and scientific professions need to continue basic scientific research, and here we are making considerable progress. But increased concern with prevention will also have a decided impact on how primary-care doctors practice medicine. With a shift to health-based rather than morbidity-based medicine, the role of the "new physician" includes a healthy dose of patient education.

Second, practitioners of the social and behavioral sciences—psychologists, economists, and city planners along with lawyers, business leaders, and government officials—must solve the practical and ethical dilemmas confronting us: poverty, crime, civil rights, literacy, education, employment, housing, sanitation, environmental protection, health-care delivery systems, and so forth. All of these issues affect public health.

Third is the public at large. We consider this group to be important in any movement. Fourth, and the linchpin in this effort, is the public health profession: doctors, epidemiologists, teachers—who must harness the professional expertise of the first two groups and the common sense and cooperation of the third: the public. They must define the problems statistically and qualitatively and then help set priorities for finding solutions.

To a very large extent, improving health statistics is the responsiblity of every individual. So let's consider more specifically what the role of the individual should be and why health education is so important. First, and most obviously, individuals can protect themselves from illness and injury and thus minimize the need for professional medical care. They can eat a nutritious diet; get adequate exercise; avoid tobacco, alcohol, and drugs; and take prudent steps to avoid accidents. The proverbial "apple a day keeps the doctor away" is not so far from the truth, after all.

Second, individuals should actively participate in their own medical care. They should schedule regular medical and dental checkups. If an illness or injury develops, they should know when to treat themselves and when to seek professional help. To gain the maximum benefit from any medical treatment, individuals must become partners in treatment. For instance, they should understand the effects and side effects of medications. I counsel young physicians that there is no such thing as too much information when talking with patients. But the corollary is the patient must know enough about the nuts and bolts of the healing process to understand what the doctor is telling him or her. That responsibility is at least partially the patient's.

Education is equally necessary for us to understand the ethical and public policy issues in health care today. Sometimes individuals will encounter these issues in making decisions about their own treatment or that of family members. Other citizens may encounter them as jurors in medical malpractice cases. But we all become involved, indirectly, when we elect our public officials, from school board members to the president. Should surrogate parenting be legal? To what extent is drug testing desirable, legal, or necessary? Should there be public funding for family planning, hospitals, various types of medical research, and medical care for the indigent? How should we allocate scant technological resources, such as kidney dialysis and organ transplants? What is the proper role of government in protecting the rights of patients?

What are the broad goals of public health in the United States today? The Public Health Service has defined these goals in terms of mortality, education, and health improvement. It identified 15 major concerns: controlling high blood pressure, improving family planning, pregnancy care and infant health, increasing the rate of immunization, controlling sexually transmitted diseases, controlling the presence of toxic agents or radiation in the environment, improving occupational safety and health, preventing accidents, promoting water fluoridation and dental health, controlling infectious diseases, decreasing smoking, decreasing alcohol and drug abuse, improving nutrition, promoting physical fitness and exercise, and controlling stress and violent behavior. Great progress has been made in many of these areas. For example, the report *Health, United States, 1998* indicates that in general, the workplace is safer today than it was a decade ago. Between 1980 and 1993, the overall death rate from occupational injuries dropped 45 percent to 4.2 deaths per 100,000 workers.

For healthy adolescents and young adults (ages 15 to 24), the specific goal defined by the Public Health Service was a 20% reduction in deaths, with a special focus on motor vehicle injuries as well as alcohol and drug abuse. For adults (ages 25 to 64), the aim was 25% fewer deaths, with a concentration on heart attacks, strokes, and cancers. In the 1999 National Drug Control Strategy, the White House Office of National Drug Control Policy echoed the Congressional goal of reducing drug use by 50 percent in the coming decade.

Smoking is perhaps the best example of how individual behavior can have a direct impact on health. Today cigarette smoking is recognized as the most important single preventable cause of death in our society. It is responsible for more cancers and more cancer deaths than any other known agent; is a prime risk factor for heart and blood vessel disease, chronic bronchitis, and emphysema; and is a frequent cause of complications in pregnancies and of babies born prematurely, underweight, or with potentially fatal respiratory and cardiovascular problems.

Since the release of the Surgeon General's first report on smoking in 1964, the proportion of adult smokers has declined substantially, from 43% in 1965 to 30.5% in 1985. The rate of cigarette smoking among adults declined from 1974 to 1995, but rates of decline were greater among the more educated. Since 1965, more than 50 million people have quit smoking. Although the rate of adult smoking has decreased, children and teenagers are smoking more. Researchers have also noted a disturbing correlation between underage smoking of cigarettes and later use of cocaine and heroin. Although there is still much work to be done if we are to become a "smoke free society," it is heartening to note that public health and public education efforts—such as warnings on cigarette packages, bans on broadcast advertising, removal of billboards advertising cigarettes, and anti-drug youth campaigns in the media— have already had significant effects.

In 1997, the first leveling off of drug use since 1992 was found in eighth graders, with marijuana use in the past month declining to 10 percent. The percentage of eighth graders who drink alcohol or smoke cigarettes also decreased slightly in 1997. In 1994 and 1995, there were more than 142,000 cocaine-related emergency-room episodes per year, the highest number ever reported since these events were tracked starting in 1978. Illegal drugs present a serious threat to Americans who use these drugs. Addiction is a chronic, relapsing disease that changes the chemistry of the brain in harmful ways. The abuse of inhalants and solvents found in legal products like hair spray, paint thinner, and industrial cleaners—called "huffing" (through the mouth) or "sniffing" (through the nose)—has come to public attention in recent years. *The National Household Survey on Drug Abuse* discovered that among youngsters ages 12 to 17, this dangerous practice doubled between 1991 and 1996 from 10.3 percent to 21 percent. An alarming large number of children died the very first time they tried inhalants, which can also cause brain damage or injure other vital organs.

Another threat to public health comes from firearm injuries. Fortunately, the number of such assaults declined between 1993 and 1996. Nevertheless, excessive violence in our culture—as depicted in the mass media—may have contributed to the random shootings at Columbine High School in Littleton, Colorado, and elsewhere. The government and private citizens are rethinking how to reduce the fascination with violence so that America can become a safer, healthier place to live.

The "smart money" is on improving health care for everyone. Only recently did we realize that the gap between the "haves" and "have-nots" had a significant health component. One more reason to invest in education is that schooling produces better health.

In 1835, Alexis de Tocqueville, a French visitor to America, wrote, "In America, the passion for physical well-being is general." Today, as then, health and fitness are front-page items. But with the greater scientific and technological resources now available to us, we are in a far stronger position to make good health care available to everyone. With the greater technological threats to us as we approach the 21st century, the need to do so is more urgent than ever before. Comprehensive information about basic biology, preventative medicine, medical and surgical treatments, and related ethical and public policy issues can help you arm yourself with adequate knowledge to be healthy throughout life.

FOREWORD

Sandra Thurman, Director, Office of National AIDS Policy, The White House

A hundred years ago, an era was marked by discovery, invention, and the infinite possibilities of progress. Nothing peaked society's curiosity more than the mysterious workings of the human body. They poked and prodded, experimented with new remedies and discarded old ones, increased longevity and reduced death rates. But not even the most enterprising minds of the day could have dreamed of the advancements that would soon become our shared reality. Could they have envisioned that we would vaccinate millions of children against polio? Ward off the annoyance of allergy season with a single pill? Or give life to a heart that had stopped keeping time?

As we stand on the brink of a new millennium, the progress made during the last hundred years is indeed staggering. And we continue to push forward every minute of every day. We now exist in a working global community, blasting through cyber-space at the speed of light, sharing knowledge and up-to-the-minute technology. We are in a unique position to benefit from the world's rich fabric of traditional healing practices while continuing to explore advances in modern medicine. In the halls of our medical schools, tomorrow's healers are learning to appreciate the complexities of our whole person. We are not only keeping people alive, we are keeping them well.

Although we deserve to rejoice in our progress, we must also remember that our health remains a complex web. Our world changes with each step forward and we are continuously faced with new threats to our well-being. The air we breathe has become polluted, the water tainted, and new killers have emerged to challenge us in ways we are just beginning to understand. AIDS, in particular, continues to tighten its grip on America's most fragile communities, and place our next generation in jeopardy.

Facing these new challenges will require us to find inventive ways to stay healthy. We already know the dangers of alcohol, smoking and drug abuse. We also understand the benefits of early detection for illnesses like cancer and heart disease, two areas where scientists have made significant in-roads to treatment. We have become a well-informed society, and with that information comes a renewed emphasis on preventative care and a sense of personal responsibility to care for both ourselves and those who need our help.

Read. Re-read. Study. Explore the amazing working machine that is the human body. Share with your friends and your families what you have learned. It is up to all of us living together as a community to care for our well-being, and to continue working for a healthier quality of life.

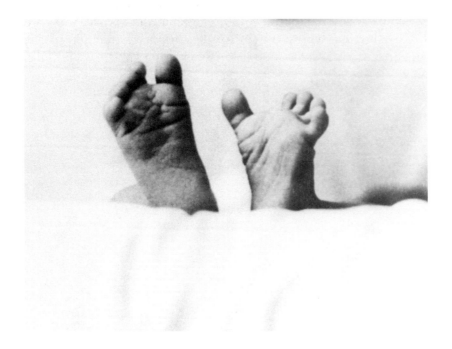

*The history of the nine months preceding . . . birth would prob-
ably be far more interesting and contain events of greater moment than all the threescore and ten years that follow it.*

—*Samuel Taylor Coleridge*

Pregnancy and childbirth are normal occurrences, not medical illnesses. Throughout the history of the human race, women have
borne children in a process that—step-by-step, cell-by-cell—has
not changed over the centuries. But our understanding of the process
has grown and, consequently, has made the experience of pregnancy
richer than ever before.

Pregnancy is more than a biological process. It is an experience that profoundly changes a woman both physically and psychologically and deeply affects her partner and their relationship. Becoming parents exposes men and women to emotions and experiences that no one can anticipate or appreciate without living through them.

Today's parents-to-be are generally luckier than their counterparts in the past. The medical risks of having a baby are lower than ever. The ability to diagnose potential problems and treat them before birth is greater than before; the options for choosing birth attendants, locations, and approaches to labor and delivery are more varied.

Yet an important link connects present and past and also explains the dramatic evolution of childbirth and infant care. That link is supplied by the family—mother, father, and child—who grow and learn together during the most exalted of human experiences.

1

AN ANCIENT AWE

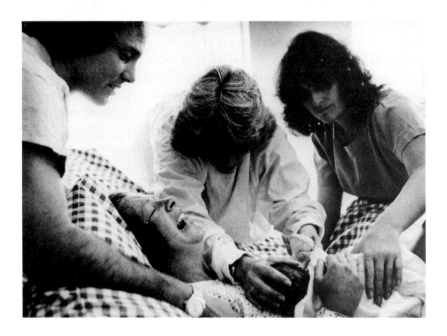

Throughout history childbirth has been regarded as one of the most mysterious processes of life. Primitive people with no knowledge of physiology (the way the body works) or anatomy (the structure of the body) often did not relate sex to pregnancy or birth. These people believed women were impregnated by spirits that dwelled in food, water, or air. Pregnant women were not considered to be delicate or ill but were expected to continue with their regular chores—stopping only for a short time to give birth, often alone and out in the open—and resuming their work once again.

Centuries later, pregnant women were given special care but still did not have the technology or resources that are available today. Babies were brought into the world not by physicians but by midwives (women trained and experienced in childbirth matters). Unfortunately, these women usually could do little to assist mothers when the labor was difficult. In some early societies, the midwife pressed down or even sat on the pregnant woman's stomach to aid in delivery. Among the Mandingo tribe in Africa, the midwife lifted a woman in labor onto her back and walked around with her, shaking and rolling her from side to side to force the baby out of the womb.

In ancient Egypt, expectant mothers prayed for assistance from various goddesses, such as Bes, protector of childbirth, and Hat Hor, patron of pregnant women. Egyptian women sat on birth stools during delivery and were attended by four midwives. In the city of Saïs, site of the first known medical school, courses in midwifery were taught by female physicians.

In ancient China women squatted during labor and were attended by midwives who had no training at all. They used dried herbs, applied topically, to control bleeding and a boy's urine mixed with vinegar sprinkled onto hot bricks for the mother to inhale in order to speed up labor. Not surprisingly, the death rate was very high—for mothers and infants alike.

In India, Hindu women about to give birth entered a clean hut where they ate gruel or inhaled smoke from the blackened skin of snakes to hasten labor (this method, however, was not in the least bit effective). The new mothers could "lie in" for as many as 10 days before finally returning to their usual responsibilities.

Ancient civilizations developed some of the same procedures used today to handle difficult births. The first cesarean delivery, or surgical removal of a fetus from the abdomen, is believed to have occurred in Greece in the 13th century B.C. And according to the Roman poet Ovid, the god Apollo removed his child Aesculapius by cesarean from the womb of Coronis after she betrayed him. Another version of the myth is that Coronis had contracted a severe infection and raging fever, and that the baby was removed from her uterus shortly before she died.

The Greek Hippocrates (460–377 B.C.), widely considered the father of medicine, taught that pregnancy could not continue for more than 300 days. Thereafter the baby would become hungry and start moving violently in order to rupture the membranes of the womb and begin the mother's labor.

The Greeks had two different types of midwife: ordinary midwives who handled most deliveries, and senior midwives—what we today call doctor-midwives—who prescribed drugs and induced labor prematurely. Senior midwives also intoned hymns to the birth goddesses, Artemis, Hera, and Eileithyia. This practice was followed by the women of ancient Rome, who prayed to the goddess of labor, Lucina. Roman women also used birth stools for delivery, a method favored by Herophilus in the book he wrote on midwifery in 300 B.C.

After the fall of the Roman Empire, in the 5th century A.D., medical advances ground to a halt. A book dating from the 11th century recommended a very primitive approach to difficult labor: placing the woman on a sheet held at the corners by four strong men, who shook the sheet vigorously by pulling on opposite corners until the woman gave birth.

The next two and a half centuries ushered in a more scientific interest in fetal development. During this time the German philosopher and scientist Albertus Magnus wrote that a fetus became very active during its seventh month in the womb, rested in the eighth month, and came into the world at the end of the ninth month healthy and strong. If the child was born during the eighth month, it would be too exhausted to survive.

During the Renaissance (1450–1600), midwives continued to perform deliveries, and male physicians were banned from taking part. According to legend, a German physician who disguised himself as a woman was discovered at a delivery and burned at the stake. Superstitions about birth were widespread. Multiple births were considered punishment for sexual misconduct— adultery or intercourse with animals or even the devil.

By the 16th century, midwives began to receive formal instruction, and men began to enter the field. For the first time cesarean sections were performed on living women, although the mortality rate for the mothers was almost 100%. Birth stools remained popular, and snuff, or sneezing powder, was used to speed up labor or expulsion of the placenta.

During this era, forceps—devices that aid in the delivery of a baby through the birth canal—were developed, and midwives and physicians used various techniques to turn a baby who was in the breech position (feetfirst in the womb) to make delivery easier and safer.

Women giving birth during the 16th century were aided by midwives and used birthing stools during delivery.

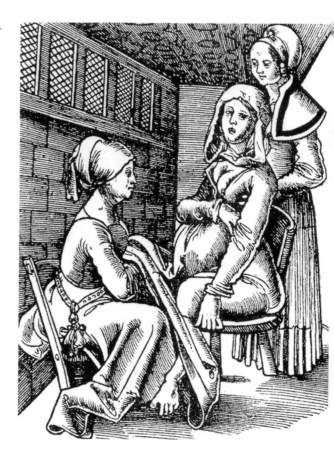

In the 17th century, scientific thought generally held that babies made their way into the world through their own exertions, as a baby chick pecks through the shell of its egg. The outstanding French obstetrician of the 17th century, François Mauriceau, was the first to rupture the membranes of the amniotic sac to induce labor and to control bleeding from a misplaced placenta. Mauriceau was also the first physician to substitute the bed for the birth stool. Not until the end of the 19th century, however, did the delivery table replace the bed.

In the 18th century, it became more common for men to undertake obstetrics. They were often required to tie the corners of a blanket around their necks so they could deliver a baby by touch but not actually see what was happening. At the same time, obstetricians improved their skills at using various forceps to help in difficult deliveries; a few also succeeded in performing cesarean sections in which both mother and child survived.

Major advances occurred in the 19th century. One was the use of anesthesia, introduced to women in childbirth in 1847 by a British physician, James Young Simpson. He used chloroform, a powerful liquid that produced strong fumes that patients inhaled during difficult deliveries. In the mid-1800s, obstetrician Ignaz Semmelweis discovered that there was a correlation between the number of new mothers who died from infection and those who had been examined by physicians directly after they had performed autopsies on fever victims. Semmelweis realized that germs were being carried to these mothers by their doctors and insisted that the doctors wash their hands before attending to the women.

Unfortunately, Semmelweis's discovery was ridiculed by most of his colleagues, and Semmelweis himself was dismissed as a crank. But his findings were confirmed by the renowned French experimenter Louis Pasteur, whose discovery of bacteria as a source of infection took place

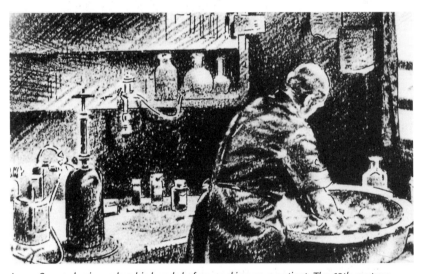

Ignaz Semmelweis washes his hands before working on a patient. The 19th-century physician recognized the importance of cleanliness in combating infections that killed millions of women in childbirth.

in the mid-1800s. His findings confirmed Semmelweis's theory, and soon obstetricians stepped up their efforts to prevent infection in childbirth, primarily by using clean linens and washing their hands. Once this became a regular practice, the mortality rate among mothers dropped drastically.

Another important advance was the growing ability of physicians to control infection and bleeding, which vastly increased the survival rate for mothers undergoing cesarean deliveries. The first successful cesarean delivery in the United States was performed in 1876, by an Ohio physician who used a pocketknife to operate on a woman lying on a kitchen table. The mother recovered fully.

The 20th century brought major advances in surgical anesthesia and infection control. Doctors replaced chloroform with safer agents, such as gas-ether. Morphine and scopolamine, powerful sedatives, came into use in the early 1900s; these drugs induced a "twilight sleep" in which a woman was barely aware of what was going on around her. The use of antibiotics and the ability to perform blood transfusions also helped improve the safety of cesarean deliveries.

Today much has changed, and yet much remains the same. "Birthing chairs"—modern-day descendants of the ancient birthing stools—are gaining in popularity. Nurse-midwives, combining up-to-date medical knowledge with an age-old sense of the human dimensions of birth, are delivering more babies. Obstetrics involves more "high-technology," but childbirth remains a "high-touch" experience. Science has demystified many of the processes by which a fetus develops and a child enters the world, but the birth of a human being continues to inspire a timeless awe and appreciation for the complexity of life.

2

A LIFE BEGINS

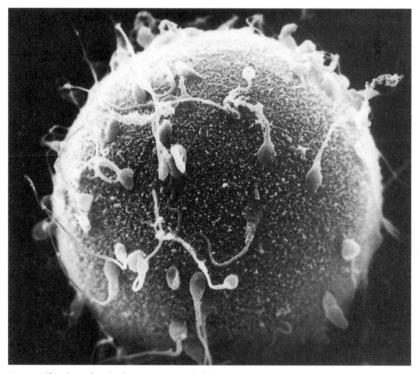

A magnification of a single egg surrounded by sperm.

L ife starts with a dance—a swirl of sperm surrounding a single egg. No one can pinpoint the exact moment at which a single sperm from the father and an egg from the mother combine to begin the long, intricate process of forming a child. We do, however, know a great deal about what happens from that time until the moment, nine months later, when a baby enters the world.

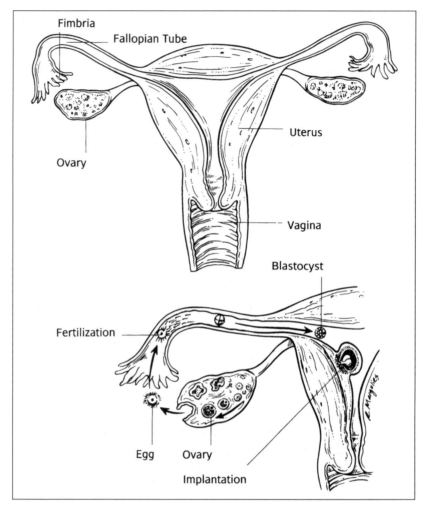

Figure 1: Above: *The female reproductive system.* Below right: *The sperm penetrates the egg in the fallopian tube, and then the fertilized egg travels to the uterus, where implantation takes place.*

CONCEPTION

The creation of sperm, regulated by hormones, begins at puberty. A single male ejaculation can contain up to 500 million sperm, all designed to fertilize a single egg (or ovum). Each of the bulbheaded sperm released into the vagina during intercourse moves on its own, propelling itself toward its target.

Nearly every sperm produced by a man in his lifetime fails to reach its mark. To succeed, the sperm must survive the acidic secretions of the vaginal canal and reach the uterus. From there it must travel up one of the fallopian tubes. If a sperm meets the ripe egg and succeeds in merging with it, fertilization occurs.

Far fewer human eggs are produced than sperm. Each woman is born with the precursors of her lifetime's supply; a total of 300 to 500 mature eggs will eventually leave the ovaries. Each month, in one or the other of the woman's ovaries, an egg is released in a process called ovulation.

This egg is then swept through the fallopian tubes to the uterus, a journey that lasts three to four days. An unfertilized egg lives for about 24 to 36 hours and then disintegrates. It is expelled during menstruation along with the uterine lining, which had prepared itself for possible pregnancy.

If a sperm, which can survive in the female two to five days, meets a ripe egg in one of the fallopian tubes, one barrier remains between them: the layer of cells surrounding the egg. Each sperm that touches the egg deposits an enzyme that dissolves part of this membrane. If a sperm encounters a bare spot, it can penetrate this barrier and fertilize the egg.

Fertilization occurs in the upper part of the fallopian tube. As the fertilized egg finishes its trip down the fallopian tube, it divides to form a tiny clump of cells. The cells become smaller with each division, so the total cell unit stays about the same size as the original fertilized ovum—smaller than the head of a pin. When it reaches the uterus, about a week after ovulation, the cell cluster burrows into the lining, a process called implantation.

THE FIRST TRIMESTER

Once nestled into the spongy uterine lining, the embryo, as it is now called, takes on an elongated shape, rounded at one end. A sac (the amnion) envelops it. As water and other small molecules cross the amniotic membrane, the embryo floats freely in the absorbed fluid, cushioned from shocks and bumps.

A primitive placenta begins to supply the growing baby with food, water, and nutrients from the mother's bloodstream and to carry waste

A human embryo lies encased in the protective sac known as the amnion. Fluid within the amnion cushions the developing embryo against external shocks.

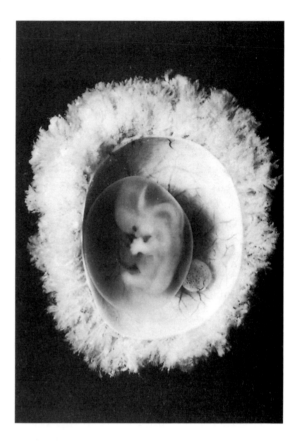

back to the mother's body for disposal. The placenta serves as a combination of lungs, kidneys, and digestive system for the baby. For the mother, it produces estrogen and progesterone, the hormones that regulate physiological changes during pregnancy.

At the end of its first month, the embryo is a little more than a quarter of an inch long—10,000 times its original size—and develops with amazing speed. Its cells differentiate into layers, tissues, and organs, grouping themselves according to the directions encoded in the genes, the parts of the cell that store inherited characteristics. The neural tube, the beginning of the nervous system, remains open. There are gill-like arches that will develop into a mouth, lower jaw, and throat. Beneath them is a tiny U-shaped tube that will form a heart.

In the second month, the sculpting of the face begins. Two tiny folds of tissue appear on either side of the head; they will later develop into ears. There is a tiny depression where the nose will be and a thickening that will become the tongue.

The head, larger than the rest of the body, seems to rest on the chest as if it were too heavy to hold up. The brain develops rapidly, and its various sections, nerves, and membranes begin to grow. Cartilage spreads upward to enclose it, although the skull will not knit firmly together for almost a decade, when the brain finally stops increasing in size. In medical terms, the embryo becomes a fetus.

By the end of the third month, the fetus is completely formed. Its heart beats rapidly. Its face is modeled into a unique configuration of features. The fetus can open its mouth, squint, and purse its lips. The "buds" for its limbs have developed into arms and legs, and fingers and toes have been defined. The fetus begins to exercise its muscles and to move freely within its fluid-filled capsule, but its mother cannot yet detect any signs of activity. Sexual organs appear, as well as all other major internal organs.

THE SECOND TRIMESTER

The fetus grows rapidly in its fourth month, stretching to a length of more than six inches and reaching the weight of five ounces. It begins to drink some of the amniotic fluid, which its kidneys process and pass back into the amniotic sac as urine. Its heartbeat can be heard through a special stethoscope. A temporary covering of hair grows on its eyebrows, palms, soles, and upper lip. Its skeleton develops, with bone cells filling in and hardening the cartilage molds.

In its fifth month, a fine down called *lanugo* (from the Latin for wool) covers its body. Most of this silky covering will rub off by the time of birth. The eyes open and close. The ears are sensitive enough to detect sounds. Nails appear on the fingers and toes, and the ridges on the palms and soles are fully formed. The fetus begins testing its reflexes, grasping and sucking as well as kicking and moving. It still has plenty of room for somersaulting, but its mother now can feel the twists and turns and detect a daily pattern of activity and rest.

By the end of the sixth month, the fetus is 13 inches long. Although its vital organs are quite well developed, its lungs are not yet mature. If it were born at this time, it might not survive because it cannot breathe on its own.

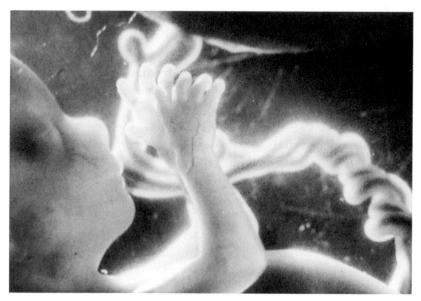

The umbilical cord is clearly visible in this photograph of a four-month-old fetus. The cord connects the fetus with the food and oxygen passed through the placenta.

A protective coating, called *vernix,* forms over the *lanugo,* clinging to the hairy parts and creases of the body. The skin, once the color of old parchment, begins to look more opaque but remains very wrinkled. The fetus looks more like a tiny old person than the fat babies that appear in diaper commercials.

THE THIRD TRIMESTER

In the last trimester, the fetus adds inches and pounds to its frame. Much of the weight is deposited under the skin as fat. This fat layer will provide necessary energy during birth and help maintain body temperature afterward. Gradually the fetus takes on a more "babylike" appearance, with pinkish skin and chubby limbs.

In the last weeks in the womb, the lungs produce a crucial material that lines the small air sacs. This substance, *surfactant,* will help the baby breathe on its own. In preparation for breathing, the fetus spends about half of the time making respiration-like movements.

By the end of the eighth month, the fetus probably will adopt the typical head-down, or *vertex,* position in the mother's pearshaped womb. If it does not, the baby is then said to be in a *breech* position, which means it may be feet- or buttocks-down. When this occurs, the obstetrician may attempt to turn the baby inside the mother's womb, or may consider alternate methods of delivery.

In the ninth month, the baby's head moves lower into the mother's pelvis, like an egg settling into an egg cup. Rather than moving its entire body, the fetus prods the mother with an arm or a leg.

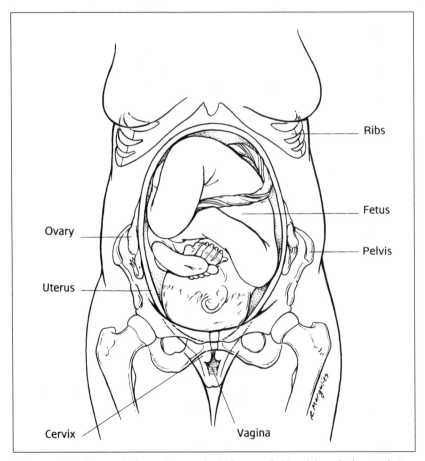

Figure 2: *This diagram depicts a nine-month-old fetus nestled head down in the womb. By the eighth month of development most fetuses adopt this position, which facilitates childbirth.*

INFERTILITY

Infertility afflicts many American couples. Twenty percent of all newlyweds are unable to conceive a child, and 10% of all couples who have children are unable to have any more. In about 90% of the cases, physicians can determine a specific cause. Abnormal menstrual patterns, suppression of ovulation, blocked fallopian tubes, and uterine fibroids (benign growths) can prevent women from becoming pregnant. A low supply of sperm, poor quality sperm that tends to be sluggish, malformed, or travel in the wrong direction, and difficulty or inability to ejaculate are common reasons why men cannot impregnate women.

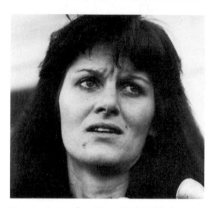

Surrogate mother Mary Beth Whitehead made news in 1987 when she fought to keep a baby she had conceived via artificial insemination. The court decided in favor of the man who had hired Whitehead to bear his child.

In some cases, drugs can correct the problem and allow couples to conceive. Many of these drugs, however, cause the release of more than one egg from the woman's ovaries and may result in multiple births. Another treatment for infertility is the fertility pump, which injects a synthetic hormone into a woman's arm through a needle inserted into her vein. The hormone then triggers ovulation.

Other treatments for infertility include microsurgery (often with lasers) to open blocked egg and sperm ducts and sound waves that monitor ovulation and the effects various drugs have on the ovaries. There is even a home ovulation kit that allows couples to pinpoint ovulation with extreme accuracy. Apart from these treatments are several remarkable and sometimes quite controversial methods for conceiving or having a baby. These include the following:

- Artificial insemination: In this, the oldest alternative to conventional conception, a man's sperm is injected into a woman's vagina and conception then continues along normal lines. Newer techniques allow for the selection of only the most active sperm for insemination.

- In vitro fertilization: This technique involves removing an egg cell from the mother (usually with a long needle) and mixing it with the father's sperm in a lab dish for a specific time period. If the fertilized egg cell shows signs of developing, it is returned to the woman's uterus within several days by means of a hollow tube inserted through the vagina and cervix and into the uterus. The egg then implants itself in the lining of the uterus and the pregnancy continues as normal. Conceived by in vitro fertilization, Louise Brown, the world's first "test tube" baby, was born in England on July 25, 1978. The success rate of in vitro fertilization varies greatly but is estimated at about 20%. The cost of each attempt is approximately $10,000.

- Embryo transfer: This is a method by which the sperm of an infertile woman's husband is placed in another woman's uterus during ovulation. Five days later, the fertilized egg is transferred to the man's wife, who then carries it to term. Embryos may also be frozen for later implantation in a process called cryopreservation, which is highly controversial because of legal issues concerning the "ownership" of the unborn child. The first baby developed from a frozen embryo was born in Australia in 1984.

- Gamete intra-fallopian transfer (GIFT): This method involves placing sperm and an egg into the fallopian tubes to imitate normal development. Less time-consuming than in vitro fertilization, GIFT allows the fertilized egg to travel on its own through the fallopian tubes and become implanted in the uterus. The success rate of this method is 20% to 30%.

- Host Uterus: In this procedure, the sperm from a man and the egg from a woman are combined in a lab dish and then implanted in a second woman. This woman agrees to bear the child, who is not genetically related to her, and to give it up after birth for a fee.

- Surrogacy: Surrogates are women who agree to be artificially inseminated with the sperm from an infertile woman's husband and to carry the baby to term. The surrogate usually receives a fee for the baby, whom she must give up after delivery. The widely publicized and highly controversial "Baby M" case, in which a surrogate mother fought to keep the child, raised many legal and ethical issues, some of them as yet unresolved. Paid surrogacy has been declared illegal in New Jersey (where the Baby M case occurred), a decision many observers believe will set the precedent for other states.

In addition to the foregoing options, infertile couples also may look to adopt—become legally responsible for the care and upbringing of a child who has been either orphaned or given up by its parents. Children of all ages are available for adoption, and couples interested in exploring this option should contact either state or local agencies for more information.

Nine months after the ovum was fertilized by the sperm, the process of fetal development, growth, and maturation is complete. Two cells have grown to 6,000 billion. A heart has been working for months. A brain is responding to stimuli. Arms and legs have grown, and a face has formed with a set of features that will distinguish this child from all others. In the darkness of the womb, waiting to be born, lies a unique individual, ready to journey into the world.

3

NINE MONTHS OF CHANGE

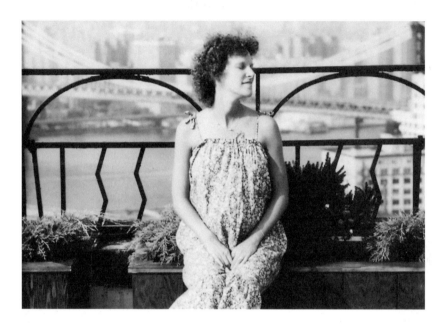

Pregnancy is a time of constant change for the mother-to-be. As her child develops, her body adapts to its unspoken needs, transforming the way she looks and feels. The father, too, goes through many stages as he prepares for his new role and responsibilities.

THE FIRST TRIMESTER

Some women do not need to be told they are pregnant: Their bodies give them the first clues. The uterus retains its lining, rather than shedding it as usually happens in a menstrual period.

Many women use home pregnancy tests, which, although they are quick and private, are inaccurate about 15% of the time. Blood tests performed in a doctor's office are far more reliable.

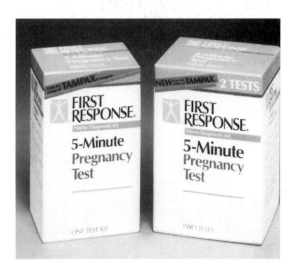

Some women experience light spotting instead of a normal period, but most miss their period entirely.

In addition, they may feel a fullness in their breasts, an uneasiness in their stomachs, and overwhelming fatigue late in the day. Some of the changes resemble those many women experience before a period, but they are more intense and persistent.

Millions of women use home pregnancy tests to find out if they are, indeed, pregnant. These tests detect human chorionic gonadotropin (HCG), a chemical messenger produced only during pregnancy, in a woman's urine. Less sensitive than blood tests available at a clinic or doctor's office, home pregnancy tests vary in their reliability. If the woman carefully follows the instructions, she can usually detect a pregnancy within three to nine days after an expected menstrual period. Some tests even claim to be able to detect a pregnancy one day after a missed period.

The biggest drawback of home pregnancy tests is a high "false negative" rate: About 10% of women whose tests indicate they are not pregnant actually are. In another 5% of women, the tests show that they are pregnant when they are not.

During the first trimester, the high levels of HCG characteristic of early pregnancy may trigger morning nausea and vomiting; some women find that nibbling on crackers or dry toast before slowly getting out of bed helps them overcome this. In addition, rising levels of the hormones progesterone and estrogen produce changes in the milk glands and ducts in the breasts; consequently, the breasts may increase in size and feel tender. The pressure of the growing uterus against the bladder causes the woman to urinate more often. But for many women, the first trimester brings only slight variations in the way they normally feel and act.

THE SECOND TRIMESTER

The midtrimester—the fourth through the sixth month of pregnancy—is usually a quiet time for the mother. Many women feel more energetic than before, but the transformation of their bodies becomes much more noticeable.

The expectant mother's waistline disappears; her breasts grow fuller; her belly becomes round and firm. Pregnancy hormones cause changes in skin pigment, darkening the skin around the nipples, the areola, and the *linea alba,* a white line—unnoticed by most people—that runs down the abdomen to the pubic bone. In pregnancy, it becomes a dark line, or *linea nigra,* but lightens again after delivery. Sometimes the pigment on a woman's face also darkens in a masklike pattern. Vaginal secretions, perspiration, and saliva increase.

Many women develop yearnings for odd foods—not just the pickles and ice cream of popular lore but also exotic dishes they may never have liked before. No one understands precisely why women crave certain foods during pregnancy, but some scientists speculate that hormones may change their taste perceptions, leading some women to find familiar foods repulsive and new ones enticing.

By the end of the sixth month, the uterus increases its weight by 20 times. The production of blood cells in the mother's body accelerates; total blood volume increases by 30% to 50%. The heart, working harder to pump the greater supply of blood, enlarges slightly and shifts position. By midpregnancy the breasts, functionally ready for nursing, secrete a thin amber or yellow substance called *colostrum.*

For the mother, the most exciting experience of the midtrimester is feeling the baby moving inside the womb, an event that usually happens between the 16th and 22nd weeks. At first, most mothers sense only gentle swimming sensations. As the baby grows, however, they feel stronger pokes and prods.

A pregnant woman feels the life stirring within her. A fetus usually begins moving in its mother's womb during the fourth month of development.

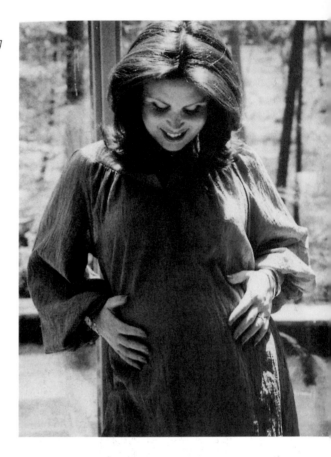

THE THIRD TRIMESTER

During the final three months of pregnancy, the growing uterus pushes against the lungs, and even though the rib cage now expands to take in more oxygen than before, many women feel breathless after any exertion. When a woman sits or lies down for a prolonged period of time, the physical pressure of the growing uterus on the vessels that carry blood to and from the lower limbs makes it harder for them to empty. A woman's legs and ankles can become swollen if she spends too many hours on her feet; such swelling, called *edema,* can also be the result of fluid retention. Also, as the uterus squeezes against the stomach, digestive acid may be pushed into the esophagus, causing heartburn.

In the ninth month, the baby "drops" or settles low in the pelvis, making breathing much easier. Some women feel tired, especially if the need to urinate frequently or the baby's kicks keep them awake at night. Many mothers-to-be look forward to delivery with both apprehension and eagerness, waiting restlessly for the day when they can hold their babies for the first time.

THE MOTHER'S FEELINGS

Being pregnant changes the way a woman thinks about herself and the world. A woman carrying a baby she has longed to have, supported by a loving partner and facing no medical risks, may feel a deeper sense of happiness than she has ever known. If the circumstances of her pregnancy are less than ideal, however, she may struggle against troubling anxieties.

At some stage of her pregnancy, almost every mother worries whether her baby will be normal and healthy. She can find assurance if she has regular prenatal care, discusses any concerns with the obstetrician or midwife, and develops healthy habits—if, in other words, she does everything possible to ensure that her baby will get a good start in life. Many women also worry about their appearance—weight gain, diminished attractiveness—and suffer minor physical discomforts. Talking to other pregnant women or to new mothers can help a woman keep her perspective.

Women who are in their first pregnancies are usually apprehensive about labor and delivery. They wonder how they will cope with the pain or with emergencies. Many women and their spouses attend childbirth classes that provide useful information and prepare both partners for every step of the childbirth process. Couples who gain some knowledge about the situation feel less anxious, although unspoken worries besiege all new parents.

The physiological changes of pregnancy affect a woman's mood. In early pregnancy, many women feel weepy, irritable, and emotional—somewhat as they may feel just before their menstrual periods. As the pregnancy progresses, many feel calmer and more energetic, although some seem touchier than usual or more vulnerable to intense emotional outbursts throughout pregnancy. These feelings are normal and should be expressed, not bottled up.

Despite the inevitable worries, many women consider pregnancy one of the most glorious times of their life. Some feel tuned in to the creative energies of their bodies. Some glow with the excitement of being, as one woman interviewed put it, "full of life." As women approach delivery, they are usually eager to see and hold the child they have carried inside them so long.

THE FATHER'S PERSPECTIVE

When a couple has been planning or hoping for pregnancy, the father's immediate reaction is to feel enormous pride at siring a child. Soon, however, he may feel overwhelmed by the sudden weight of responsibility. Many men begin to question their own ability as providers and doubt whether they can furnish the stability a child needs. Others feel left out or unneeded, as the mother-to-be becomes the center of attention, even though their emotional support is more crucial than ever before. Many fathers worry about their wife's well-being or fear that the baby will not be healthy or normal. Such concerns are normal, and often talking them over with the obstetrician or midwife can help men overcome unnecessary anxiety.

During pregnancy, some men may experience a change in their feelings for their partner. Some husbands are almost overly protective, yet they also may feel confused or put off if their wife seems more tired or testy than usual. Some think their wife has never been more attractive; others are put off by her bulging belly. And sex becomes an issue. The husband may fear that having sex will hurt his wife or the growing baby, although unless a woman develops complications or has been expressly warned to refrain from having sex to prevent a miscarriage, most couples can safely continue to have intercourse throughout pregnancy.

For most men, the pregnancy becomes real when, laying their hand on their wife's abdomen, they feel the baby move for the first time. From that moment on, many men picture themselves as fathers and envision the unborn baby as a child with whom they will talk and play.

Although a man may try his best to offer support to his partner, he may suffer tension as he relives his feelings about his own childhood. The best way to come to terms with this is by talking about it. Partners who work through such issues are prepared to support each other after the baby is born and to deal with the challenges of becoming parents. By the final trimester, most have had time to resolve their doubts and allay their fears.

An increasing number of men are taking a much more active role in preparing for the birth of their children. Some fathers-to-be attend birthing classes with their wives and participate as "coaches" during labor. Many are present at the moment their baby enters the world and share the exultation of becoming part of a new family.

THE PARENTS-TO-BE

Ideally, a couple can share the small joys that abound throughout the pregnancy. They can also prepare for the birth by taking childbirth classes and by working together on the nursery. The worry about labor and delivery is offset by the intense anticipation of the new life that will enrich their own.

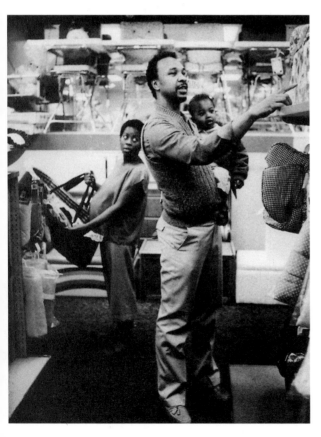

Accompanied by one child—with another on the way—a couple shops for their nursery. The physical and emotional rigors of pregnancy can strain relationships, but it is also a time of expectation and excitement.

Many men and women on the verge of becoming parents feel a great need for parenting themselves. The mother-to-be may turn to her partner for affection and reassurance. He may try to meet her needs while contending with his own doubts and mixed feelings. Yet if both care about each other's expectations and anxieties, they may find themselves closer than ever as they count down to the day of their child's birth.

The nine months of waiting are, in short, as crucial for the new parents as they are for the unborn child. During the time the infant is preparing for life, his or her parents are preparing for the most demanding and rewarding roles of their own lives—those of mother and father.

4

PRENATAL CARE

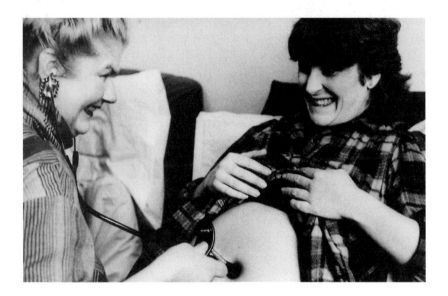

A pregnant woman has to take good care of herself in order to provide good care for her unborn child. This means that she must have regular medical checkups, eat properly, exercise safely, be sure to get extra rest, and avoid potential threats to the baby's well-being.

PRENATAL CARE

Women should make their first prenatal visit as soon as they discover they are pregnant. From that point on, most women see their obstetricians or nurse-midwives once a month until the 28th week of pregnancy. Some women schedule these visits at the birthing center where they plan to deliver their baby. Others visit the obstetric clinics at local medical centers.

At every visit, a woman can expect the doctor or nurse-midwife to check her weight, blood pressure, urine (for sugar and protein, signs of diabetes, or other medical conditions), and hands and feet for swelling, or edema. The physician also inquires about any symptoms that may indicate there is a problem with the pregnancy. Beginning at about the third month, the health care provider listens for the fetal heartbeat through a special stethoscope (a fetoscope), feels the shape of the uterus by gently pressing on the abdomen, and measures the height of the uterus, or *fundus*.

As they enter the last trimester, women see their doctor or midwife every other week until the 36th week, then weekly until labor begins. During these visits, the health care provider checks the baby's estimated size, presentation (whether the baby's head, feet, or bottom is first), and, as the woman approaches the end of pregnancy, examines her cervix to see if it has begun to thin (efface) or to open up (dilate).

These checkups provide information about how the baby is growing. A woman's weight and fundal height should steadily increase. If they do not, and if her blood pressure is high or if she has sugar or protein in her urine, she may need to undergo tests to determine whether the baby's well-being or her own health is at risk.

NUTRITION

The National Research Council recommends that the mother gain between 25 and 30 pounds during pregnancy. If she gains substantially less, the risk to the infant is high. One of the largest threats to a developing fetus as well as to a newborn infant is lack of proper nutrition or low birth weight.

Because a well-balanced diet is critical for the baby's health both before and after birth, the American College of Obstetricians and Gynecologists has developed the following dietary guidelines for mothers-to-be:

- Expect to consume about 300 more calories a day than before pregnancy.

- Do not restrict salt. (In the past, doctors commonly feared that salt led to fluid retention and swelling of the hands or feet. Most doctors now think that only excessive salt intake is potentially dangerous.)

- Drink six to eight glasses of liquids each day, including water, fruit and vegetable juices, and milk.

- Concentrate on eating the right foods, not on weight watching.

- Never diet during pregnancy.

- Eat four or more servings each day from these food groups: fruits and vegetables; whole grain or enriched bread and cereal; and milk and milk products. Eat at least three servings of meat, poultry, eggs, fish, nuts, or beans.

Many pregnant women also take vitamin supplements, though none can replace or equal the benefits of a well-balanced diet. Most prenatal vitamin compounds include calcium, vitamin A, vitamin D, and vitamin C. Many obstetricians contend that the only supplements needed in pregnancy are a B vitamin called folic acid (0.3 mg daily) and iron (30 to 60 mg daily).

Large doses of certain vitamins can be dangerous, however. Excessive vitamin A, which can be obtained in adequate amounts from green and yellow vegetables, can cause severe birth defects. High doses of vitamin D, which can be obtained in adequate amounts from fortified whole or skim milk, have also been linked with fetal malformations.

EXERCISE

Early in the 20th century, many pregnant women were treated like fragile invalids, forced to spend most of their pregnancy in bed. Today, physicians recommend that women remain active throughout pregnancy. Regular exercise (three times a week) is better, safer, and more effective than occasional workouts.

Some pregnant women swim, ski, play tennis, and even run marathons, but pregnancy is not a good time to take up such strenuous sports. As their breasts and bellies grow, some women may find vigorous exercise uncomfortable; physicians recommend brisk walks as a good alternative.

Guidelines of the American College of Obstetricians and Gynecologists for exercise by low-risk pregnant women who have checked with

Women participate in a special aerobics class designed for mothers-to-be. Once considered dangerous, mild-to-moderate exercise for pregnant women is now often recommended by health professionals.

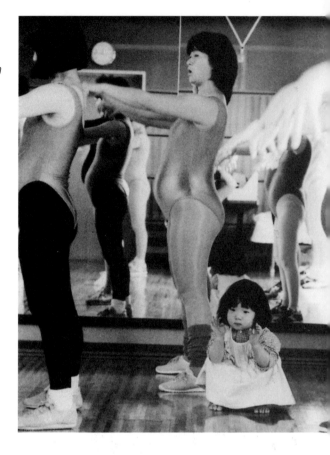

their health care provider to make sure that they can continue their exercise programs include:

- You can continue to exercise and derive health benefits even from mild-to-moderate exercise routines. Regular exercise (at least three times a week) is preferable to more intermittent activity.

- Avoid exercising on your back after the first trimester. Also avoid prolonged periods of motionless standing. Both positions can reduce blood flow to the uterus.

- Be aware that you have less oxygen available for exercise. Stop exercising when you become fatigued, and do not exercise to exhaustion.

- Avoid exercises in which a loss of balance could be harmful. Also avoid any exercises that could cause even mild trauma to the abdomen.

- Avoid overheating, especially in the first trimester. Drink plenty of fluids before and during exercise, wear layers of "breathable" clothing, do not exercise on hot, humid days, and avoid immersing yourself in a hot tub or sauna.

REST AND WORK

Rest is as important as exercise, and the woman who is not used to taking naps may have to schedule rest periods. If insomnia or the frequent need for urination during the night become a problem, daytime catnaps may be the answer. Under no circumstances should a pregnant woman take sleeping pills or any other medication to help her sleep, nor should she take any other medication without first consulting her physician.

Many women continue working outside the home until the final weeks of pregnancy. The best guide to how long to continue is the woman's own sense of energy and comfort. Being on her feet for long periods of time may cause discomfort. Women with other children at home may also want extra help with their daily tasks during the final weeks of pregnancy.

A TEENAGE MOTHER'S SPECIAL NEEDS

Although most mothers-to-be can follow the same set of general guidelines and often have very similar needs, pregnant teens require different care—psychological and physiological—and frequently have a very different set of needs. Although pregnancy rates among teens have declined since the 1980s, the United States continues to have the highest rates of adolescent pregnancy of any developed country. Each year close to 1 million American teenagers become pregnant.

The Alan Guttmacher Institute, a family planning organization headquartered in New York City, has released statistics comparing the incidence of teen pregnancies in the United States with other countries. In the United States, for every 1,000 teenage women between 15 and 19 years of age in 1981, there were 96 pregnancies and 54 births.

This contrasts with 45 pregnancies and 31 births in England and Wales; 44 pregnancies and 28 births in Canada; 43 pregnancies and 25 births in France; and 35 pregnancies and 16 births in Sweden.

In the United States, four out of every five teenage girls who become pregnant are unmarried; 30,000 are under age 15. More than four out of 10 teenage girls become pregnant at least once before they reach age 20. Of those teenagers who do become pregnant, 45% undergo abortions. Nearly one-third of the abortions performed in this country are performed on teenagers, who are less likely to have abortions early in pregnancy, when the operation is safer. Of the teenagers who continue their pregnancies, more than 90% keep their babies.

Although the teenage birth rate has declined in recent years, the number of births by teenagers has increased because the number of teenagers in the population has increased. The largest decline in teenage pregnancy was found among black teens. Smaller declines were found for non-Hispanic white teens, while the rates for Hispanic teens rose slightly.

Researchers have linked teenage pregnancy with earlier *menarche* (onset of menstruation) and increased sexual activity. In a Johns Hopkins University survey of urban adolescents, the mean age for first intercourse was 16.2 years for girls and 15.7 for boys. Many adolescents either are unsure how to use birth control or simply do not even try. In one survey of sexually active girls between ages 15 and 19, only 65% always used birth control; 25% used it occasionally; and 10% used none at all.

Many teens do not obtain contraceptives—or information about them—because they feel ambivalent about becoming or being sexually active. As one sociologist put it, "Many teenagers can reconcile their sexual activity only if it's spontaneous or unplanned."

Some teens choose to become pregnant in order to cure feelings of loneliness, helplessness, or insignificance. For such teens, pregnancy seems a way of asserting their independence or of declaring themselves their mother's equal. Others become pregnant to keep a boyfriend or to impress their friends. Tragically, most have not thought through the implications of having and caring for a child.

Pregnancy itself poses health risks for the teen mother-to-be and her baby, especially if the mother is under 15 years of age. According to the American College of Obstetricians and Gynecologists, teenage mothers are more likely than adult women to develop complications in pregnancy, and their child is more likely to have a low birth weight (less than 5.5 pounds) and to die in its first year of life.

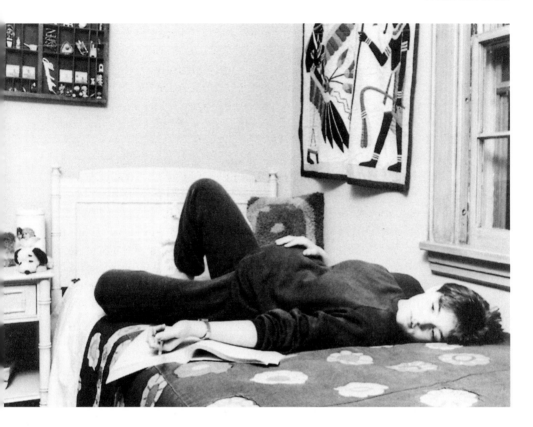

Pregnant and unmarried, an adolescent contemplates her future. Many teenage girls who become pregnant are physically and emotionally unprepared for what lies ahead.

Many of these medical risks can be reduced by prenatal care. According to a study done by the National Institute of Child Health and Human Development, pregnant teenagers who receive adequate prenatal care gain more weight during pregnancy and deliver fewer premature or underweight babies.

Yet nearly one in 10 pregnant adolescents neglects to start prenatal care until the third trimester or receives none at all. As a group, children whose mothers were age 17 or less when they were born tend to have more difficulties in school and poorer health than children whose mothers were older when they were born.

Pregnancy has other effects on a teenager's life. Adolescents who give birth before completing high school are less likely to obtain a degree and more likely to get pregnant again. Without education, these teens can become trapped in poverty. Two-thirds of the families headed by a mother age 14 to 25 live below the poverty level.

Women who were teenage mothers are more likely to be unemployed or to have lower-paying jobs. They also have higher rates of separation, divorce, and remarriage. Sadly, their children are more likely to become pregnant as teenagers as well. In one study, 82% of girls who give birth at age 15 or younger are daughters of teenage mothers.

In the past most programs addressing teen pregnancy were aimed at adolescents who were already pregnant or had given birth. Today, the emphasis has shifted to prevention, especially to the issue of birth control, a topic on which many teenagers are alarmingly uneducated. Many young women fail to use contraceptives, for instance, in the mistaken assumption that they cannot become pregnant the first time they have sex or if they have it very infrequently.

Because teens often know so little about pregnancy and birth, many European countries, particularly in Scandinavia, educate children about sex at an early age, usually around age seven; and every child has received some instruction in conception and contraception by age 12. In Sweden, for example, children are taught the basics of human physiology and biology by the time they are seven or eight, and the facts about contraception by the time they are 10 or 12. Largely as a result of this nationwide sex education, there are only 35 teen pregnancies per 1,000 teenage women in Sweden.

The United States lags behind Europe, but some strides have been made. The state of Wisconsin has set up a pioneer program designed to deal with the issue of teenage pregnancy. The state's Abortion Prevention and Family Responsibility Act of 1985 provides for sex education in public schools, counseling programs for teens, abortions without the need for parental consent, and a state adoption center. The law also holds the parents of teenagers who have babies legally responsible for those children "so far as the parent is able" and the teenager is not.

The National Campaign to Prevent Teen Pregnancy was founded in 1996 to raise awareness of the problem of teenage pregnancy, provide assistance to those working in the field, and help resolve the religious, cultural, and public values differences that surround the problem.

IF THEY'RE OLD ENOUGH TO GET PREGNANT, THEY'RE OLD ENOUGH NOT TO.

There's a forty percent chance she'll get pregnant before she's nineteen. One of the million teens who get pregnant each year.

That's the highest teen pregnancy rate in the industrialized world. And you don't have to look far for the reason: two-thirds of sexually-active teens in America use no method of birth control or fail to use it consistently.

The personal consequences of teen pregnancy are tragic and the social costs are staggering. Over $16 billion each year. That's the price we pay for misinformation and ignorance about the facts of life.

We need to equip our children with basic information about the risks of pregnancy and about contraception.

Most teens know less about such things than you might think. Few people realize that only two states and the District of Columbia require sex education programs in schools. And the mass media, marketing sex with no mention of precautions, only make matters worse.

Even parents who care the most may fail to make sure their children are informed—fearing they might appear to condone behavior they wish to discourage. But research shows that when parents hesitate, teens tend not to.

Studies also find that teens who've been thoroughly informed about the facts of life are much more likely to say no to peer pressure. And to start later.

That's why Planned Parenthood encourages better parent-child communication. Works to improve sex education. And maintains that all sexually-active people, including teens, should be able to get the birth control help they need and want.

Given the facts, teens can make responsible decisions. Denied the facts, all they can make are mistakes.

Biologically, after all, any teenage girl *can* get pregnant. The only question is whether she won't.

You can help. Write us for more information. Use the coupon.

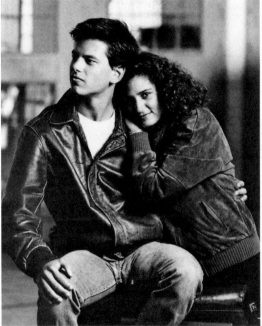

Teen pregnancy is everybody's problem. I want to help:

☐ Please send me information about Planned Parenthood's POWER (Parents Organized to Win Educational Rights) Campaign so I can make a difference where I live.

☐ Send me a copy of the booklet, "How to Talk with Your Child about Sexuality" (one dollar enclosed).

☐ Here's my tax-deductible contribution to support all of Planned Parenthood's programs encouraging responsible decisions by teens and adults: ☐ $25 ☐ $35 ☐ $50 ☐ $75 ☐ $150 ☐ $500 or: $_____.
Send your check to 810 Seventh Avenue, New York, NY 10019

NAME _____

STREET/CITY/ZIP _____

Planned Parenthood®
Federation of America

An uninformed approach to sexuality and birth control can saddle young people with the large responsibility of caring for a child. In the United States one million teenage girls become pregnant each year.

SMOKING

Smoking endangers two lives: the mother's and her unborn baby's. It boosts the likelihood of miscarriage, fetal distress, stillbirth, low birth weight, heart defects, premature birth, and impaired growth. There is a direct correlation between the number of cigarettes smoked daily and the likelihood of having short, underweight, or small-headed infants. Babies born to women who smoke often have bronchitis and asthma. Studies reported by the American Council on Drug Education have tied smoking to reduced fertility in men and women; others have linked it to cleft palate, a birth defect in which the roof of the mouth is abnormally formed, and to eye malformations in babies.

Smoking increases blood levels of carbon monoxide, which impairs the fetus's oxygen supply. Cutting back or, preferably, quitting can minimize the dangers to the baby. The sooner the mother stops smoking, the better are the baby's chances of growing to a normal weight for its gestational age. Passive smoking—inhalation of other people's smoke—can also prove hazardous for an expectant mother and her baby.

ALCOHOL

More than two out of every 1,000 babies in the United States is born with a cluster of physical and mental defects called fetal alcohol syndrome. An unknown number of babies whose mothers drink while pregnant suffer from low birth weight, irritability as newborns, and various complications of pregnancy.

Alcohol is particularly dangerous during pregnancy because it crosses the placenta and reaches concentrations in the unborn baby's blood as high as in the mother's. The risk of fetal alcohol syndrome is greatest if a mother drinks three or more ounces of pure alcohol (the equivalent of six or seven cocktails) a day. Milder forms of this problem occur in about 10% of babies whose mothers consume one to two ounces of alcohol (two to four cocktails) a day.

Fetal alcohol syndrome can be prevented. The National Institute on Alcohol Abuse and Alcoholism and the U.S. surgeon general advise pregnant women—and those trying to become pregnant—not to drink at all. The only way to avoid all the potential dangers is to avoid alcohol.

CAFFEINE

Caffeine belongs to a chemical family called the xanthines, which include the compounds found in chocolate, cocoa, coffee, and black tea. Whenever a pregnant woman drinks or eats a substance containing xanthines, her baby is exposed to the same amount.

A Yale University study of 3,135 women found that women who consumed more than 150 mg of caffeine a day (a cup of coffee can have anywhere from 29 to 176 mg; a 12-ounce cola, 32 to 65 mg) suffered almost twice as many miscarriages as women consuming less or none. Caffeine has caused birth defects in laboratory rats; it is not known if it has the same effect on human beings.

MEDICATIONS

Pregnant women should consult their physician before taking any medication—prescription or nonprescription. Even aspirin, one of the most widely used drugs, can create problems if taken in large doses in the last trimester, when it may prolong pregnancy and labor, increase fetal and maternal bleeding at delivery, and interfere with fetal blood circulation.

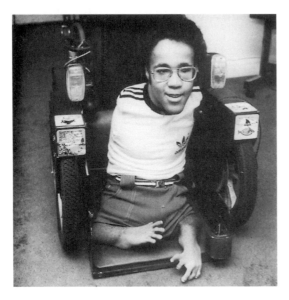

A severely deformed 18 year old operates a specially designed wheelchair. Unaware that thalidomide could cause birth defects, his mother took the prescription drug while she was pregnant with him.

The Food and Drug Administration (FDA) classifies all prescription medications according to their potential danger to a fetus. Only those in Category A, such as penicillin and its derivatives, have undergone extensive testing to prove that they have little potential for harming a fetus. Some drugs may be necessary to the mother's survival but may still threaten the health of her unborn child. Examples include certain antidepressants, which have been linked with central nervous system and limb defects, and insulin, which may play a role in skeletal malformations. In cases in which the mother's health depends on medication, doctors will try to use the lowest dose of the safest drug for the shortest possible time.

The greatest danger from drugs occurs in the first trimester, when the fetus's major organ systems are forming. In the 1950s a number of pregnant women in England took a medication called thalidomide for morning sickness. As a result, many of their children were born completely without—or with badly deformed—arms, hands, legs, or feet.

Some medications are dangerous throughout pregnancy. Tetracycline, a common antibiotic used to treat bacterial infections, has been shown to retard limb growth in premature babies and to stain permanently the teeth of children whose mothers took the drug in late pregnancy.

Sometimes the risk of drugs in pregnancy does not become obvious for years. In the 1940s and 1950s, thousands of pregnant women were given a hormone called diethylstilbestrol (DES) to prevent miscarriage. Many of their children were born with malformations of the genitals or reproductive tract that have made it difficult for them to conceive children or carry them to term. They also face an increased risk of developing cancer of the vagina and cervix.

ILLEGAL DRUGS

"Street" drugs have not been as extensively researched as medications. However, there is convincing evidence that they are extremely dangerous to the mother and, especially, to her developing child. Drug use may produce birth defects and lead to "neurochemical" birth defects (changes in brain chemistry) by disrupting normal development of the brain. Physicians urge prospective mothers to stay drug free for at least three months before they conceive as well as throughout their entire pregnancy.

Cocaine is especially dangerous for pregnant women and their babies. It can cause miscarriages, developmental disorders, and life-threatening complications during birth, such as respiratory arrest in the infant. Dr. Ira Chasnoff of Northwestern Memorial Hospital in Chicago conducted a study that compared 28 women who used cocaine while pregnant with women who did not use the drug and with women who used narcotics (any one of a group of drugs that has a sedating or depressing effect, including heroin). The cocaine users were more likely to miscarry in the first three months of pregnancy than the narcotic users.

Infants born to cocaine users often suffer major complications, including withdrawal and permanent disabilities. Because cocaine produces dramatic fluctuations in blood pressure, it can deprive a fetal brain of oxygen or cause brain vessels to burst, the prenatal equivalent of a stroke, which can cause permanent physical and mental damage.

Cocaine babies have higher rates than normal of respiratory and kidney troubles and may be at greater risk of sudden infant death syndrome

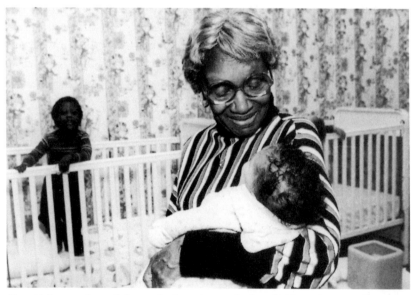

Clara Hale cares for an infant at the foster home she founded for youngsters born to addicts. Drugs taken during pregnancy can adversely affect the physical and mental capacities of a woman's unborn child.

(SIDS). This tragic affliction strikes infants unexpectedly, causing them to stop breathing and often die. Visual problems, lack of coordination, and developmental retardation are also common in children born to cocaine users. They tend to feed poorly, sleep irregularly, suffer from diarrhea, and show marked irritability and increased respiratory and heart rates.

Babies born to women who abused sedatives, such as barbiturates, during pregnancy may be physically dependent on the drugs and develop breathing problems, feeding difficulties, disturbed sleep, sweating, irritability, and fever. Barbiturates can cross through the placenta easily and cause birth defects and behavioral problems.

Marijuana smokers have smaller, sicker babies and a higher risk of stillbirths, according to the book *Normal and Problem Pregnancies*. Based on a study of 1,690 mother-child pairs in Boston, there is good evidence that the use of marijuana in pregnancy can lower birth weight and cause abnormalities similar to those of fetal alcohol syndrome. The women who smoked marijuana while pregnant were five times more likely than the others to have babies with problems such as small head size, irritability, and poor growth.

RADIATION AND OTHER ENVIRONMENTAL RISKS

High levels of radiation of the type used for cancer therapy have been associated with defects. Diagnostic X-rays are not a significant threat, particularly after the first trimester, because they involve low levels of radiation. The Committee on Radiology of the American Academy of Pediatrics says that because the possibility of birth defects resulting from X-rays is extremely low, even abdominal X-ray examinations should be performed if genuinely needed during pregnancy.

Dental X-rays, which use extremely low radiation directed at the mouth, are not considered hazardous. Most dentists routinely use lead shields that block any X-rays from reaching a patient's major organs.

Few scientific data are available on fetal vulnerability to pollutants, toxic wastes, heavy metals, pesticides, gases, and synthetic compounds. Some studies indicate that lead and cadmium are hazardous to a fetus, that pesticides such as DDT can be found in the breast milk of women living near sprayed areas, and that exposure to certain chemicals may increase the risk of birth defects.

5

PRENATAL TESTING

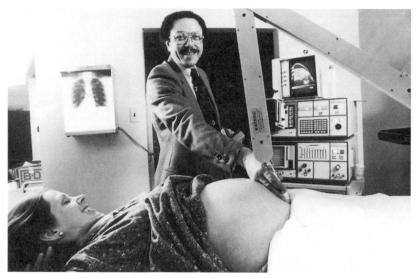

Ultrasound examination.

I s my baby all right? It is the question asked by every mother-to-be as she yearns for reassurance that her child will be healthy. Today, prenatal tests can reveal more about a fetus than once was thought possible, and increasing numbers of babies undergo their first physical exams before birth.

ULTRASOUND (SONAROGRAPHY)

Ultrasound is a procedure in which high-frequency sound waves (those too high-pitched to fall within the normal range of hearing) are bounced off structures within the womb, producing echoes that can be converted into images on a display screen.

Ultrasound is of great use to physicians. It can establish exactly how far along a woman's pregnancy is—crucial information in timing other tests and delivery; reveal if the mother is carrying more than one child; identify possible causes of vaginal bleeding; and detect serious birth defects such as *hydrocephalus* (excessive fluid within the brain), *anencephaly* (a large part of the brain missing at birth), muscular and skeletal malformations, some heart, lung, kidney, and genital tract abnormalities, and problems in the spinal cord. Ultrasound can also show whether the baby is growing as it should, whether there is too little or too much amniotic fluid, and whether the placenta is ruptured or blocking the birth canal.

Ultrasound has been used in pregnancies for 35 years with no reports of significant harmful effects. Many obstetricians use ultrasound routinely and believe it should be done at least once in every pregnancy. Others feel that it is unnecessary in normal, uncomplicated pregnancies and should only be used when a problem is suspected. It should also be remembered that no test is completely accurate, and a normal ultrasound scan doesn't guarantee that the baby will be normal.

ALPHA-FETOPROTEIN (AFP) SCREENING

Alpha-fetoprotein (AFP) screening can be used on pregnant women between the 16th and 18th weeks of pregnancy. It tests the mother's blood for the presence of a crucial protein manufactured mainly in the liver of a fetus. An abnormally high or low quantity of the protein can indicate problems with the unborn child.

A high AFP level in the blood may indicate neural tube defects—a sign that the brain or part of the spinal cord will not form normally—or malformations in the abdominal wall. Some of these problems are fatal; others can be surgically corrected after birth. In order to confirm the presence of a defect, physicians may call for further tests with high-resolution ultrasound or for the measurement of AFP levels in the amniotic fluid. Even if the test discloses no defects, an elevated AFP can indicate increased risk of premature delivery, low birth weight, or other complications that can surface at a later stage of the pregnancy.

Low AFP levels can signal serious chromosomal disorders. Normally, each human cell contains 46 chromosomes, the 23 pairs of rodlike structures within the nucleus of the cell that carry the genes. Children afflicted with Down's syndrome—a form of mental retardation—possess 47 chromosomes. If a woman's risk of having a Down's child, based on her AFP and age, is greater than the risk of miscarriage that may be brought on after an amniocentesis, genetic testing is recommended.

AFP screening is as safe and simple as any blood test for the mother and poses no risk for the fetus. However, more than 95% of abnormal readings are "false positives"—mistaken indications of problems. These mistakes are often the result of faulty timing. If the test is performed too early in pregnancy, normal AFP levels may seem too low; if the test is performed too late, the levels may seem too high. These findings can create unnecessary anxiety and involve further tests that may pose a risk to the fetus.

GENETIC TESTING

Prenatal genetic testing can identify hundreds of hereditary diseases before birth. It is recommended for women who have had a previous child with a genetic disorder, who have a family history of hereditary illness, or who may carry X-linked disorders (such as hemophilia) that they may pass on to their sons. It is also recommended for couples who both carry a recessive trait for hereditary diseases.

One major hereditary disease is Tay-Sachs. This ailment refers to an enzyme deficiency that occurs almost exclusively among young children of eastern European Jewish ancestry. It is hard to detect because for six to nine months the infant appears normal. Thereafter, however, its development rate slackens. By the end of the first year, the child's innate and acquired skills have begun to deteriorate. The child loses mobility; speech is impaired. The child usually dies before his or her fifth birthday. One in every 30 eastern European Jews is a carrier; but because the trait is recessive, both parents must carry it for their child to be affected. If both parents are carriers, the chances of their child being affected are one in four. Carriers can be identified by a blood test.

Because the risk of chromosomal defects increases with the mother's age, genetic counselors have recommended testing for all women over the age of 35. The two types of genetic tests used most frequently are *chorionic villi sampling* and *amniocentesis*.

A family meets with genetic counselors to discuss hereditary patterns and their possible impact on future offspring. Prenatal testing is often recommended if a family has a history of genetic disorders.

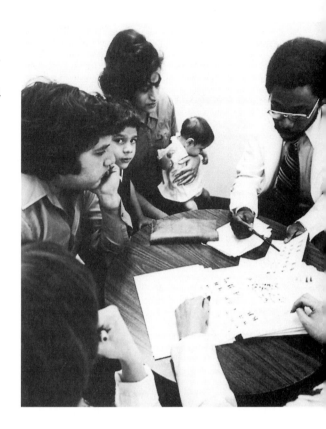

Chorionic Villi Sampling (CVS)

Chorionic villi sampling, a relatively new test for genetic defects, is performed between the 10th and 12th weeks of pregnancy. A physician uses a syringe or hollow tube to remove a small sample of the chorionic villi (the tissue surrounding the fetus).

The chromosomes in the fetal cells are then analyzed in the laboratory for evidence of serious genetic disorders, including Down's syndrome; Tay-Sachs and other metabolic disorders in which a crucial enzyme is missing (such as galactosemia and Hunter syndrome); and disorders of the blood cells (such as sickle-cell anemia and hemophilia). Test results are available within a week, early enough for a first-trimester abortion if the fetus has a major disorder and the parents decide not to continue the pregnancy. CVS cannot, however, detect neural tube defects.

One drawback to CVS is that it may cause a miscarriage. Some test centers report that one of every 200 women who undergo the test miscarries; others report even higher miscarriage rates. In unusual cases, CVS results may not be clear-cut, and the woman may have to undergo amniocentesis to get more precise information.

AMNIOCENTESIS

In amniocentesis, performed during the 15th to 17th week of pregnancy, an obstetrician, guided by ultrasound, removes about three tablespoons of amniotic fluid through a thin needle inserted in the abdomen. Fetal cells from the fluid are then grown in a specially prepared culture, a process that takes several weeks. Once the cells are grown, laboratory technicians can examine the chromosomes under a microscope for signs of genetic disorders and other hereditary diseases. The major risk with amniocentesis is miscarriage, which occurs in nearly one out of every 200 women tested.

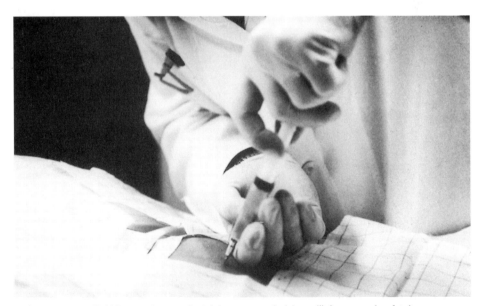

A doctor extracts fluid for amniocentesis. A laboratory technician will then examine fetal cells contained in the fluid for signs of genetic flaws and hereditary disease.

Amniocentesis is suggested for the same women who might consider CVS. Another drawback is that results are not available for several weeks. If a serious defect is found and a couple decides not to continue the pregnancy, the woman must undergo a riskier and more psychologically and physically traumatic second-trimester abortion.

Sampling of Fetal Blood or Skin

A few rare but devastating hereditary diseases can be detected only by analyzing blood or skin from the fetus. Fetal blood cells can show if the baby has inherited some uncommon blood diseases. Skin samples can indicate rare hereditary skin diseases.

The obstetrician who takes a percutaneous umbilical blood sampling (PUBS) uses high-resolution ultrasound to guide a needle directly into the umbilical cord to obtain a blood sample. PUBS generally has replaced fetoscopy, a test in which obstetricians insert a sort of minitelescope into the womb to guide them in removing blood cells or skin samples. Fetoscopy is used only rarely, to detect very unusual life-threatening hereditary skin conditions; it triggers miscarriage in 5% of the women who undergo testing.

TESTING A BABY'S
WELL-BEING IN THE WOMB

If a woman develops complications during pregnancy, such as high blood pressure, diabetes, or infections, or if the baby is not growing as it normally should, other prenatal tests can determine whether the baby would be safer in the womb or the outside world. These tests, performed in the last trimester, include the following:

- Fetal Movement Monitoring: In this do-it-yourself test, a woman counts how often her baby moves in a 30- or 60-minute period. If the baby does not move at least 3 times an hour or does not move at all for 12 hours, physicians can perform further tests to determine if the fetus is in jeopardy.

- Fetal Biophysical Profile: This test—performed with a sophisticated ultrasound scanner that provides moving real-time images—assesses fetal breathing, body movements, and muscle tone. It also indicates whether there is too much amniotic fluid, a condition called hydramnios, which is most likely to develop if a woman is carrying twins or has diabetes or Rh-incompatibility. Too little amniotic fluid—a condition known as *oligohydramnios*—may indicate a problem with the baby's kidneys or a leak in the amniotic membranes.

Based on standardized "norms," each baby receives a score between 0 and 10. Low scores indicate poor oxygen supply and potential fetal distress; high scores indicate low risk of distress before or during birth.

- Non-Stress Test: An external fetal heart monitor, strapped around the mother's belly, measures the baby's heart rate when it moves. Normally, a baby's heart rate speeds up. A minimum of 2 such accelerations in a 20-minute period indicates a healthy fetus.

- Contraction Stress Test: A fetal heart monitor measures the baby's heart rate during contractions induced either by stimulation of the mother's nipples (manually or with warm towels)

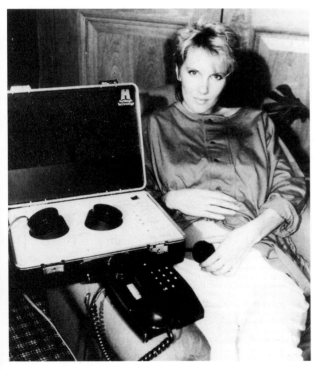

A woman operates an at home fetal monitor. This experimental machine enables mothers to record the heartbeat of a fetus and transmit the information via telephone to hospital technicians.

or by intravenous administration of oxytocin, a hormone that triggers uterine contractions. The baby's response indicates how well it may cope with the physical stress of labor and alerts doctors to potential problems during delivery.

Although in most cases testing reveals nothing more than a healthy baby, there are those cases where the pregnancy is either not progressing as it normally should or the fetus has a disease. In the next chapter we will explore the different complications and diseases that can affect the developing fetus.

6

COMPLICATIONS OF PREGNANCY

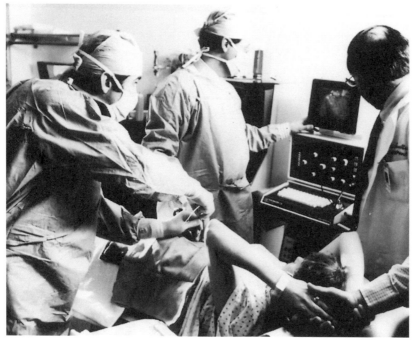

Doctors perform an in utero blood transfusion.

E ach year more than three million women in the United States give birth. Most have uneventful pregnancies, and most of their babies are born healthy. In about 15% of pregnancies, however, there is an increased risk of complications, such as maternal hypertension or impaired growth of the fetus. Indeed, in as many as 30% to 40% of all pregnancies, there is some exception to the usual course of labor and delivery.

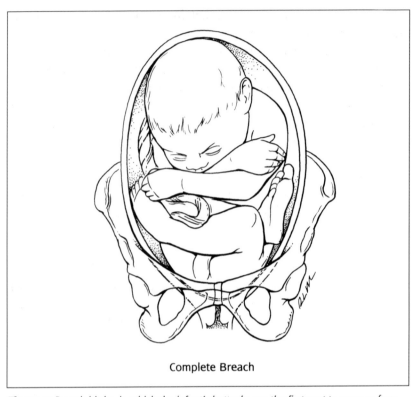

Complete Breach

Figure 3: *Breech births, in which the infant's buttocks are the first part to emerge from the mother's body, can be difficult. To facilitate delivery, a doctor may try to turn the fetus in the womb.*

ECTOPIC PREGNANCY

In an ectopic pregnancy, the fertilized egg implants itself in the fallopian tube, the abdominal cavity, the ovary, or the cervix instead of in the uterus. Tubal pregnancies are the most common. Any woman who is of childbearing age, who has had intercourse, and who feels abdominal pain with no reasonable cause may have such a misplaced pregnancy.

The incidence of ectopic pregnancies has tripled in recent years and continues to rise. The risk of ectopic pregnancy increases in women who have used intrauterine devices (IUDs) for birth control or who have pelvic inflammatory disease—a serious infection of the reproductive organs caused by IUDs—or suffer from sexually transmitted diseases. These last can cause scarring that, in turn, interferes with the passage of an egg through the fallopian tubes.

During the late 1970s there was one ectopic pregnancy for every 250 normal pregnancies; during the late 1980s the ratio was one in 70; during the late 1990s it was estimated to be as frequent as one in 40. About 50% of women who have an ectopic pregnancy are later able to have a normal pregnancy. The remainder experience another ectopic pregnancy, fail to become pregnant, or have miscarriages.

If a fertilized egg implants itself in a fallopian tube, it goes through the normal course of development. The usual signs of pregnancy may occur, and both the woman and her doctor may believe that the pregnancy is normal. But between the eighth and 12th weeks, the tube can no longer expand to accommodate the growing fetus and placenta. It then bursts.

As a result, the woman will bleed internally and feel lower abdominal pains or an ache in her shoulders as the blood flows upward toward the diaphragm. If the bleeding is great, the woman can go into shock, a condition characterized by low blood pressure and high pulse rate. Symptoms are hot and cold flashes, nausea, dizziness, fainting, pelvic pain, and irregular bleeding.

The physician usually makes an incision in the fallopian tube and removes the fetus and placenta. The tube is left open so that it will heal without making scar tissue, which could hinder or prevent later pregnancies.

MISCARRIAGE

A *miscarriage,* or spontaneous abortion, is the term used to describe a pregnancy that ends before the 20th week of gestation. About 10% to 15% of all expectant mothers miscarry each year. Approximately 95% of all miscarriages occur before the 16th week; most happen by the eighth to 10th.

Most miscarriages are chance occurrences that cannot be fully explained and do not affect a woman's ability to deliver a healthy baby at a later point in her life. An estimated 70% to 90% of all women who miscarry become pregnant again, although their chances for successful pregnancies depend on the reasons for the original miscarriage. If the cause of a miscarriage can be identified and treated—for example, a malformation of the uterus that can be corrected by surgery—the prospects of successful pregnancy are much brighter.

The most common "treatment" for a threatened miscarriage—a condition in which a woman begins spotting, cramping, or bleeding but the gestational sac has not been expelled—is rest. If the bleeding and cramping stop, the woman can get up in a few days. Usually the pregnancy continues normally.

Cases of inevitable miscarriage, a miscarriage whose progress cannot be halted, are signaled by pain and bleeding. The cervix opens, the membranes of the amniotic sac break, the uterus contracts, and the sac containing the developing embryo is expelled.

Following a miscarriage, the woman is usually bedridden for at least 48 hours. Sometimes her obstetrician will perform dilatation and curettage (D and C), stretching the cervix to permit the passage of a special type of knife to empty the uterus. If the fetus and placenta are not completely expelled, the doctor may remove them with a suction device.

Rh FACTOR

About 85% of Americans have a chemical substance in their red blood cells known as the Rh factor. People who carry it are called Rh-positive (Rh+); those who do not are Rh-negative (Rh−). Rh+ red blood cells in the bloodstream of an Rh− person stimulate the production of antibodies that react with the Rh+ blood cells and help bring about their destruction.

If a man is Rh+, his child may be Rh+. At the time of delivery (or miscarriage or abortion) of the first Rh+ baby, fetal blood cells in the placenta enter the mother's bloodstream. If the mother is Rh−, her immune system will respond by developing antibodies, specific substances produced by the body to destroy the Rh+ cells.

Because this process usually occurs at the time of birth, there is no threat to the baby in the first pregnancy. But when an Rh− woman is pregnant with a second Rh+ fetus, her Rh antibodies may cross the placenta in large numbers and reach the baby's blood, where they will react with the baby's red blood cells and cause their destruction. The damage may be so severe that the baby requires life-saving actions. Tests can determine whether there is a dangerous Rh antibody level in the mother's blood. Physicians can prevent damage by giving the baby a blood transfusion after birth or even when it is still in the uterus.

The risk increases with each pregnancy, but the antibody reaction can be prevented. If the mother receives an injection of anti-Rh antibodies (trade name RhoGAM) within 72 hours after delivery, miscarriage, or abortion, the injected antibodies will rapidly destroy any Rh+ cells from the baby so they do not prime her immune system to start producing Rh antibodies. This procedure is very effective in preventing an Rh problem in future pregnancies.

HIGH BLOOD PRESSURE

Because of the unique demands on their circulatory system, women are more likely to develop hypertension during pregnancy than at any other time. Thus, the most common medical complications that occur during pregnancy are related to the mother's high blood pressure.

Blood pressure that was abnormally high before pregnancy is likely to become more severe. In the past, medical scientists suspected that a toxin, or harmful substance, caused this difficulty and thus developed the term *toxemia.* No such culprit has ever been identified, and the term has since been discarded as misleading.

If left untreated, hypertension in pregnancy can lead to convulsive disorders—called preeclampsia and eclampsia—which threaten both the mother and her unborn baby. More frequently, hypertension slows the supply of blood to the uterus and hampers the baby's growth. Mild hypertension is not considered dangerous, but the hazards to a baby depend on how high the mother's blood pressure rises and how long it remains elevated. Proper medical care is essential.

INFECTIONS

The infectious disease most clearly linked to birth defects is *rubella* (German measles). If a woman develops this infection during pregnancy, her baby may be born with severe defects of the heart, brain, and eyes. All women should be vaccinated against this disease to protect themselves and any children they may conceive.

Another common prenatal infection is *cytomegalovirus.* In adults, this infection causes only very mild flulike symptoms, but in unborn babies it can lead to much more serious consequences including brain

A nurse takes a blood sample from an infant born with AIDS. A woman afflicted with this deadly disease has a 15–50% chance of passing it on to her baby before or during childbirth.

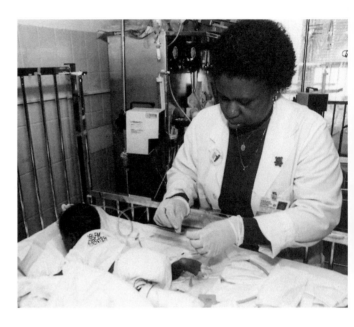

damage, retardation, liver disease, cerebral palsy, hearing problems, and other malformations. Cytomegalovirus is a common infection transmitted through any kind of close contact: kissing, breast-feeding, or sexual intercourse. There are no means of prevention other than avoiding known carriers (which is difficult because most people do not realize they are infected) and no available treatments.

Mothers with sexually transmitted diseases can transmit the infections to their babies during vaginal delivery. Such diseases include chlamydia (caused by a bacteria, a one-celled organism that can release harmful substances) and genital herpes (caused by a virus, a tiny bit of genetic material within a protein coating that invades cells and takes over their reproductive machinery so that they produce more of the virus). If these infections are transmitted, the consequences can be very serious: eye inflammation, pneumonia, damage to the nervous system, even death. If a woman develops herpes sores around the time she comes to term, her physician will deliver the baby by cesarean section to prevent a life-threatening infection in the newborn.

Acquired immune deficiency syndrome or AIDS (a fatal disease that brings about the total destruction of the body's immune system) endangers both a pregnant woman and her unborn baby. Possibly because it alters the immune system, pregnancy can precipitate or exacerbate

AIDS in a woman already infected with the human immunodeficiency virus. An infected woman's child has a 15% to 50% chance of contracting AIDS before or at birth. Babies born infected with AIDS rarely survive for more than a few years; some never become well enough to leave the hospital.

PREMATURE LABOR

Approximately 10% of all babies are born too soon. Thrust into the world before they are ready to survive on their own, they are among the most vulnerable of newborns. Obstetricians and pediatricians consider prematurity the biggest medical problem they face. In many ways, it is also the most perplexing.

Premature labor is the onset of rhythmic contractions of the uterus after the 20th week and before the 37th week of pregnancy. It results in the thinning and opening of the cervix. No one knows why nature's timetable for labor sometimes goes awry, although researchers have been investigating the phenomenon for many years. Obstetricians believe, however, that if more pregnant women seek prompt treatment it may be possible to buy more time in the womb for these babies.

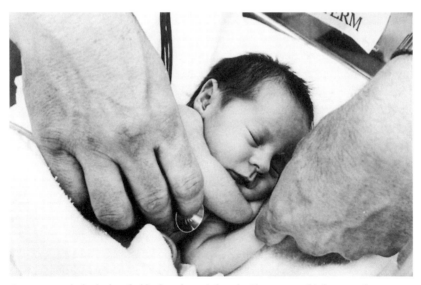

A premature baby is dwarfed by her doctor's hands. About 10% of infants are born too early, and their immature respiratory and digestive systems often require assistance.

The many warning signs of premature labor include a dull ache in the lower back; a feeling of tightness or a dragging sensation in the abdomen, somewhat similar to menstrual cramping; a sense of pressure on the lower abdomen, back, or thighs; intestinal cramps, sometimes accompanied by diarrhea; and regular tightening and relaxation of the uterine muscles.

Bed rest is the cornerstone of treatment, and obstetricians often recommend that women who develop early signs of delivering too soon should spend from several extra hours to all day in bed. If the uterine muscles continue to contract, medications are given to inhibit further progression of labor.

BIRTH DEFECTS

Major birth defects occur in two or three of every 100 births. The most common are cleft lips or palates (malformations of the lips or roof of the mouth), clubfoot (malformation of the bones of the foot), and hip dislocation (maladjustment of the bones of the hip). Despite widespread concern in recent years about the impact of environmental pollutants, there has not been a marked increase in the incidence of birth defects. Indeed, there has been a marked decline in the incidence of Down's syndrome, the most common cause of mental retardation, and neural tube defects, which result in malformations of the spinal cord, backbone, or brain. Both these disorders can be detected by prenatal tests.

If a mother is told her child is not going to be born healthy or normal according to certain medical standards, then she must consider her options. She may terminate the pregnancy if it is early enough to do so. Many mothers choose this option because they feel it is unfair to bring a child into the world to suffer.

The mother may, however, choose to continue the pregnancy and give birth to the child. This is often a painful and difficult decision to make and one that both partners must fully discuss. Caring for a handicapped child is never easy, although, over time, it can be extremely rewarding.

Many of these mothers, though, may be reluctant to risk another pregnancy, for fear that this second child will end up with the same complications. Only genetic counseling can tell for sure whether the complications were passed on or just arose as a part of that particular pregnancy. Mothers who have had previous complications should, then, check with a genetic counselor and not readily dismiss the idea of another pregnancy.

7

LABOR AND DELIVERY

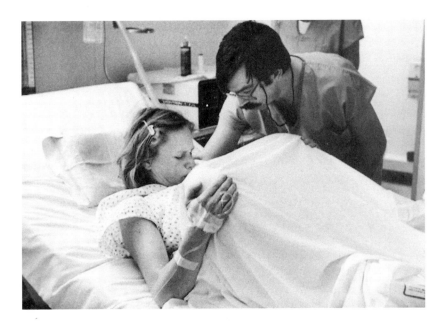

Most mothers and fathers remember their children's births as a blur of physical and emotional experiences unlike any other, but labor and delivery actually consist of a sequence of orderly stages. The more parents-to-be learn about the processes of childbirth, the better prepared they are for the unforgettable moment when their child enters the world.

THE NATURAL CHILDBIRTH MOVEMENT

Delivering a baby used to be something a doctor did in a hospital. The mother was given so many painkilling and sedating drugs that she often was barely conscious of what was happening. During the delivery, the father paced nervously in a waiting room. After its arrival, the newborn was shuttled off to the nursery, where parents could wave at it through a window.

Expectant parents, however, began to express interest in accepting less than complete medical management of birth. In the 1950s, a French obstetrician, Dr. Fernand Lamaze, developed *psychoprophylaxis*—or mind prevention—a method of easing labor pain without drugs. His techniques were described in *Thank You, Dr. Lamaze,* a book that popularized relaxation and breathing techniques in the United States. And in 1960, a nonprofit group called the American Society for Psychoprophylaxis in Obstetrics (ASPO) was formed.

At first physicians resisted this approach, but as groups for teaching pregnant women Lamaze techniques spread throughout the country, obstetricians reversed their opinion. They saw that women could indeed cope with labor without heavy medication and that their babies often developed fewer problems during and immediately after birth because they were not sluggish from the drugs given to their mothers. Today various childbirth education programs can be found in just about

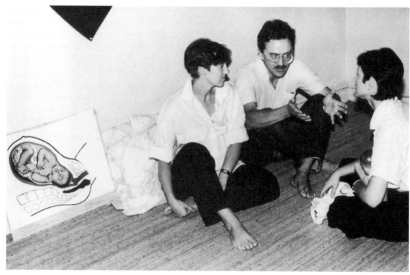

A Lamaze instructor (on right) counsels an expectant couple on natural childbirth techniques. The Lamaze method centers on alleviating labor pain with relaxation and breathing exercises.

every community in the United States. Each offers preparation for both the mother and father, enabling them to anticipate the stages of labor and to work together as a team.

Lamaze techniques have been modified over the years, but the basic theory remains the same. Rather than feeling out of control and overwhelmed in labor, a woman learns to respond to contractions by relaxing her muscles and breathing according to a prelearned pattern. The husband, her "coach" for labor, works with his wife throughout the process.

Initially, "natural" childbirth advocates opposed the use of any pain medications during labor and delivery. Today's programs are less regimented and emphasize that every woman has her own pain threshold.

CERTIFIED NURSE-MIDWIVES

For centuries lay midwives brought almost all babies into the world. Today in the United States, a modern form of midwife—the certified nurse-midwife, or CNM—has emerged as an increasingly popular alternative for parents-to-be. The 5,700 certified nurse-midwives practicing in this country deliver more than 258,000 babies a year, mostly in hospitals and birth centers.

Nurse-midwives complete standard training in nursing as well as a special postgraduate program in midwifery. They must pass qualifying examinations in order to be certified by the American College of Nurse-Midwifery. The responsibilities given nurse-midwives and the restrictions placed on them vary from state to state and, to a certain extent, from hospital to hospital. Most states require that an obstetrician be available to handle complications during labor or delivery.

For the most part, nurse-midwives handle normal pregnancies and deliveries in healthy women. They work alone, in groups, or in association with physicians, and they provide complete prenatal care; "attend," or care, for the mother throughout labor and delivery; and provide postpartum follow-up care. Many nursemidwives also provide routine gynecological care.

Lay midwives do not have formal nursing training but share the nurse-midwives' emphasis on family-centered childbirth with minimal medical intervention. Some states require lay midwives to meet certain standards to obtain licenses. In Arizona, for example, lay midwives must show evidence of training and must have observed and performed a set number of deliveries. States that do not require licensing have no such standards for lay midwives.

WHERE BABIES ARE BORN

Eventually, parents must decide where their baby will be born. There are several alternatives—as long as no medical problems develop during pregnancy or labor. For high-risk births, the best place for the baby and mother is a hospital fully equipped with special facilities, such as a neonatal intensive care nursery.

An increasing number of couples are choosing in-hospital birthing rooms. Furnished like comfortable bedrooms, these alternative settings for labor and delivery offer the best of both worlds: a low-key, family-oriented environment and immediate access to medical care in case of emergency. Some have "birthing chairs," specially molded so a woman can stay in an upright position to work with the forces of gravity in pushing her baby into the world.

Freestanding birth centers, independent of hospitals, offer a home-like setting to low-risk mothers. Their fees are lower than hospitals and their safety record is excellent. One drawback, however, is that about 10% of the mothers admitted develop complications and must be transferred to hospitals during or after delivery.

In the United States, only about 1% of babies are born at home. The American College of Obstetricians and Gynecologists opposes home births because of potential hazards to mother and child. Home-birth advocates contend that women can minimize the danger by having a qualified birth attendant on hand and by setting up a reliable procedure for rushing the mother to the hospital in case of an emergency.

COUNTING DOWN

In the final weeks of pregnancy, women notice a variety of changes—some subtle, some not. Many lose a few pounds; others experience a burst of energy or a strong nesting instinct. Among the biological signals that indicate labor may soon begin are the following:

- Engagement. In the last weeks of pregnancy, the baby's head settles into the pelvis and the mother can breathe more easily and deeply.

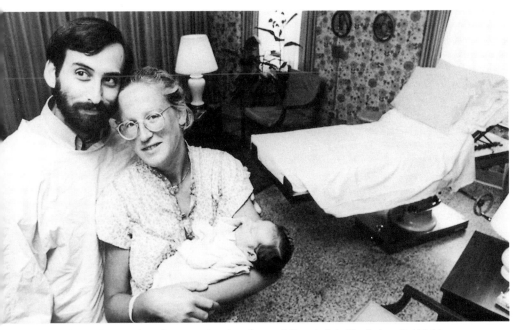

An increasing number of women are choosing to deliver their babies in hospital birthing rooms. These environments combine the comfort of a home birth with the safety of advanced medical technology.

- Brief, irregular contractions, called "Braxton Hicks" contractions—named for the British obstetrician John Braxton Hicks (1825–97), who first described their significance. The mother experiences a tightening of the abdomen. In "false" labor, contractions stop if the mother walks around, and they do not become stronger or longer.

- A "show" of pink-tinged secretions from the vagina that indicates passage of the mucous plug, which seals the uterus to protect the baby from infection.

- A trickle or gush of warm clear fluid, indicating that the amniotic sac enclosing the baby has burst. When the amniotic membranes break beforehand, labor generally begins within 24 to 48 hours. If not, the risk of infection increases because the baby is no longer protected by the amniotic sac and bacteria can travel up the vagina into the uterus.

- Regular contractions of increasing intensity. Real labor contractions often start at the back and radiate to the lower abdomen, becoming more frequent and more intense regardless of the woman's position or activity. If the baby's head is pressed against the back of the pelvis, the pain may be concentrated in the lower back.

Only a vaginal examination can determine if the cervix has begun the crucial prerequisites for delivery: effacement (thinning) and dilation (opening). Effacement is measured in percentages, dilation in centimeters or fingerwidths. In first-time mothers, effacement may occur gradually over several days; in women who have already had children, it may take only a few hours.

LABOR: THE FIRST STAGE

There are three stages of labor: The first ends when the cervix is completely dilated to 10 centimeters (or 5 fingers' width) and the baby is ready to come down the birth canal. The second culminates in the birth of the baby. The third ends with the delivery of the placenta.

The first contractions of the early or latent phase of labor are usually not uncomfortable. They last 15 to 30 seconds, recur every 15 to 30 minutes, and gradually increase in intensity and frequency. As the cervix dilates from five to eight centimeters, many women rely on breathing exercises to overcome discomfort.

The most difficult contractions come after the cervix has dilated about eight centimeters. During the last part of cervical dilation, the contractions are more painful because the woman feels greater pressure from the fetus. For first-time mothers, the first stage of labor averages 12 to 13 hours; it is much shorter in subsequent pregnancies.

PAIN RELIEF

Breathing techniques taught in childbirth classes, a massage, or a warm shower can help ease the discomfort and pain of labor.

Various analgesics (painkillers) and anesthetics can also help. The most commonly used of these include tranquilizers and barbiturates, pills given early in labor to help the mother relax; analgesics, which are injected into the blood or a muscle to relieve pain; and anesthetics, which numb the body or a particular part of the body completely.

Physicians inject narcotics by one of several methods. An *epidural block* involves insertion of an anesthetic into the membrane surrounding the spinal cord at the lower back to block sensation from the waist down. A *spinal block,* injected into the spinal canal, also numbs the lower body. A *pudendal block,* injected through the vagina, numbs the area around the vagina for an *episiotomy* (surgical enlargement of the vaginal opening to allow the baby to pass through).

The last resort is general anesthesia by means of an inhaled or injected drug that puts the mother to sleep. It is used only for emergency cesarean deliveries when there is no time to administer regional anesthetics.

All these drugs have benefits and liabilities. They can provide much-needed relief during long, hard labors, but they can also produce unwanted side effects, such as making it harder for a woman to push during the second stage or making the baby somewhat lethargic after delivery. Using pain medications is not a matter of making a right or wrong decision but of doing what suits a mother best under the unique circumstances of her baby's birth.

THE JOURNEY INTO THE WORLD

When the cervix is completely dilated, the second stage of labor begins. The baby moves into the vagina, or birth canal, and then out of the mother's body. This stage can take up to an hour or more. Strong contractions may last for 60 to 90 seconds and occur every two to three minutes. As the baby's head descends, the mother feels an urge to push. By bearing down, she helps the baby complete its passage to the outside world.

As the baby's head appears, or "crowns," the doctor makes an incision from the lower end of the vagina toward the anus to enlarge the vaginal opening. The purpose of this episiotomy is to prevent the head from causing an irregular tear in the tissue around the vaginal opening. Sometimes women can avoid an episiotomy by developing good nutritional habits throughout pregnancy, by exercising, by trying different birth positions, or by having an attendant massage the area around the vaginal opening. These methods work only if the mother's skin is elastic enough and if the baby is not exceptionally large.

Under normal circumstances, the birth of the baby is gradual: the head emerges first, then the shoulder, and then the rest. With each contraction,

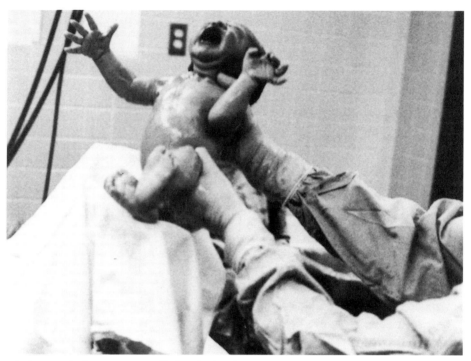

A baby utters its first cry. Most medical professionals encourage new parents to spend a great deal of time with their newborns; sometimes mother and infant even share a hospital room.

a new part is born. However, the baby can be in a more difficult position, with its head facing up rather than down and its feet or buttocks emerging first (a breech birth).

As soon as the baby is born, the obstetrician or midwife clamps the umbilical cord and suctions the baby's nose and mouth to remove amniotic fluid. Newborns undergo several routine procedures, including weight and height measurement and administration of eye drops to prevent infection caused by gonorrhea (a venereal disease). A nurse observes the infant's heart rate, breathing, muscle tone, reflexes, and complexion at one and five minutes after delivery and gives it an Apgar score—a rating scale that indicates how the baby has fared during its stressful passage—from zero to 10. Most babies score seven or higher.

In the third stage of labor, the uterus contracts firmly after delivery of the baby and, usually within five minutes, the placenta separates from the uterine wall. The woman may bear down to help expel the placenta, or the doctor may exert gentle external pressure.

If an episiotomy has been performed, the doctor sews up the incision. The uterus may be massaged, or the baby may be put to the mother's breast. Breast-feeding causes the uterus to contract and hastens its return to normal size.

CESAREAN BIRTH

In a cesarean delivery, the doctor lifts the baby out of the womb through an incision in the uterus and lower abdomen. In the United States, approximately 21% of babies were delivered by cesarean, or "c-section."

Many different circumstances may lead to a cesarean. A common one is that the mother has had a previous cesarean delivery. Fewer than 10% of women who have had a cesarean delivery have a vaginal birth with subsequent children. However, one cesarean delivery does not necessarily preclude subsequent vaginal deliveries. Some women can have a vaginal delivery—if the same complications do not develop again. If, for example, a woman's first baby was a breech baby, her second will very likely be headfirst, and she can have a normal labor and a vaginal delivery. With other problems, such as the mother's abnormally shaped pelvis, another cesarean will be necessary.

Other problems calling for a cesarean delivery are failure to progress (prolonged labor with very slow cervical dilation), signs of distress in the unborn baby, the baby's being too big to pass through the mother's pelvis, and breech presentation. Babies who are feet- or bottomfirst in the womb are often more difficult to deliver because the head is a more effective "wedge" as the baby moves through the birth canal. In addition, breech babies are more likely to be premature or smaller than average. Many twins or triplets or babies born to a woman with an unusually shaped uterus are also breech. All these factors can make a vaginal delivery especially difficult. Nevertheless, some obstetricians have had more experience in delivering breech babies vaginally and feel more comfortable with this approach if no other risks exist.

Cesareans may also be necessary because the placenta or umbilical cord is blocking the birth canal. Other problems have to do with the mother's own medical history. Diabetes, active herpes lesions, or high blood pressure can imperil the baby's oxygen supply and increase the mother's risk of a life-threatening condition called eclampsia, which is characterized by extremely high blood pressure, headaches, visual distortion and flashes, convulsions, and even coma. A final reason for a cesarean is that the baby has not grown normally in the womb or has developed problems such as Rh incompatibility, a disorder in which the mother's blood cells attack and destroy the red blood cells of her unborn baby.

In most cesareans, the mother, given a regional anesthetic, is awake and aware of what is happening, and the father can remain at her side. Once the abdomen and uterus are open, the obstetrician punctures the amniotic sac, drains off the fluid, and lifts out the baby. Usually the time from first cut to delivery is just four or five minutes; suturing then takes about 45 minutes.

Some mothers feel disappointed after a cesarean because they had hoped to have the experience of actively pushing their baby into the world. They may feel helpless, more like passive observers than active participants in their child's arrival. Or they may think that somehow they failed or did something that interfered with having a vaginal birth. Such feelings are more likely to occur if a pregnant woman has not considered the possibility of a cesarean delivery.

Most women—some sooner than others—come to terms with the circumstances and focus on the end result: a healthy baby. Whereas some feel more physical discomforts after a cesarean, such as nausea, pain, and abdominal gas, others bounce back quickly. The average hospital stay following a cesarean is three days, and the new mother must refrain from strenuous activity for several weeks.

EARLY HOURS: INTENSIVE CARING

Depending on the setting and circumstances of the birth, mothers may be able to spend almost all their time with their babies from the start. Some hospitals never separate mother and child. Others have modified lying-in arrangements that give the mother help in taking care of her baby.

Special circumstances may also keep mother and child apart. Babies with breathing problems after a cesarean delivery or a long, hard labor may remain in the nursery for several hours for observation. Some who have a low birth weight or suffered serious birth traumas may remain in the nursery for longer periods.

Three out of every 100 newborns require immediate intensive care for problems that developed before or during birth. Their best chance of survival is in a newborn intensive care nursery, which mimics the world of the womb by keeping temperature, moisture, and oxygen at an optimum level.

Premature babies often require the most and longest intensive care. Many well-equipped medical centers can save babies who were born after just 23 or 24 weeks of pregnancy instead of the normal 40 weeks. Many weigh little more than two pounds.

The major problem of the "preemie" is that all its systems are immature. The earlier the baby was born, the less well prepared its body is to survive in the world. Breathing is particularly difficult because the lungs are not fully mature until the 37th or 38th week of pregnancy. The preterm baby cannot produce surfactant, the substance that prevents the lungs from collapsing when the baby exhales, and may develop respiratory distress. To help babies breathe, a system called continuous positive

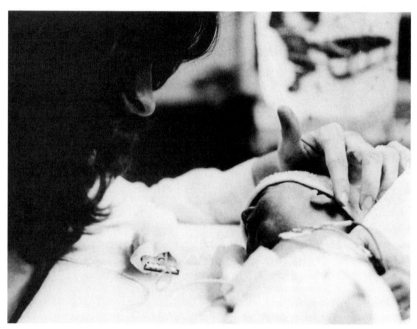

A mother visits her six-week-old son in an intensive care unit for premature babies. Modern medical technology has dramatically increased the chances of survival for prematurely born infants.

A premature infant undergoes photo-therapy in a New York City hospital. The bright lights help the child fight off jaundice, a disease caused by a build-up of a chemical called bilirubin.

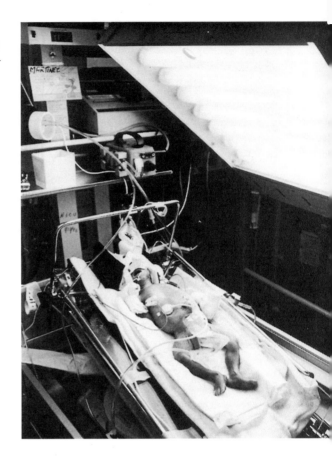

airway pressure (CPAP) provides a constant supply of pressurized oxygen administered through a tube in the windpipe.

Oxygen may increase the risk of eye damage and bring on a retinopathy of prematurity. In this disease, for unknown reasons, the blood vessels in the baby's retina, the light-sensitive tissue forming the eyeball's inner lining, grow excessively. The result can be distortion or detachment of the retina, which can eventually lead to blindness.

Preterm babies have great difficulty regulating their body temperature because they have very little body fat to insulate them. Thus, they lose heat rapidly, and the stress of being cold adds to the burden placed on their body systems. An incubator can help to maintain normal body temperature.

Feeding can also be a problem for preterm babies, who may not be strong enough to suck and swallow and who have very small stomach capacities. Their levels of blood sugar (essential for brain functioning) or calcium (essential for muscle functioning) may drop and need immediate correction. Some babies must be fed through a tube inserted through their nose that empties directly into the stomach. Very premature babies are also at risk of developing "bleeds," hemorrhages within the skull that range from minor leaks in the fluid-filled chambers of the brain to massive bleeding that causes permanent brain damage.

The length of time preemies must stay in the intensive care nursery depends on how prematurely they were born. Neonatologists—specialists in treating newborns—sometimes advise parents to expect their babies to stay in the hospital at least until the time when they should have arrived in the world.

Other babies in a newborn intensive care nursery are struggling with a range of problems. Infants who are small for their gestational age struggle to stay warm and to breathe, have low blood sugar, and suffer continued growth impairment. "Postmature" babies, who arrive after 41 weeks of pregnancy, are at greater risk because the placenta may not have been able to provide adequate nourishment and oxygen in the final weeks of pregnancy. They are more likely to inhale or ingest amniotic fluid or meconium (the name used for an unborn baby's bowel movement), and they may develop low blood sugar, temperature regulation problems, and breathing difficulties.

Babies of diabetic mothers tend to be larger than average and risk developing low blood sugar, breathing problems, tremors caused by a lack of calcium, and jaundice (the buildup of a substance called bilirubin as the baby's body breaks down its normal surplus of red blood cells).

Other high-risk newborns include those who, during birth, have suffered trauma such as fractured neck bones or skulls, bleeding within the brain, and lack of oxygen. Even babies who have not encountered problems before or during birth may develop jaundice and require "phototherapy," exposure to bright lights to clear bilirubin from their bodies.

It is difficult to predict how much time a baby must spend in an intensive care nursery. Some grow stronger and healthier every day. Others overcome one problem, such as breathing difficulties, only to encounter another, such as infection. As each day unfolds, parents ride an emotional roller coaster. Many nurseries encourage parents to spend time with their babies, holding them if possible or touching them through porthole-type openings built into the sides of the specially designed basinettes called "isolettes." Mothers often can pump their breasts to produce milk that is fed to the babies through tubes or in bottles. Often, talking to other parents with sick infants helps couples deal with their own fears.

Once high-risk infants make it over the hurdle of their shaky beginning, their futures look bright. Most babies born at risk not only survive, but thrive. Years of research have shown that the vast majority of babies requiring temporary special care develop normally in body and mind.

8

THE NEW FAMILY

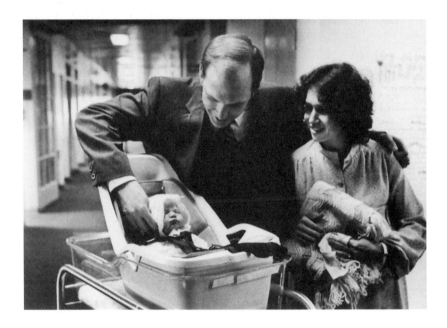

Pregnancy brings many dramatic changes for the parents. Birth brings even more. Just as understanding pregnancy and delivery helps couples through the process of bringing a new life into the world, so can anticipating and preparing for the baby's needs help the new mother and father cope better.

WHAT THE NEW MOTHER SHOULD EXPECT

Hospital stays for new mothers have been getting shorter. In 1998, maternity hospital stays averaged two days. Many hospitals offer early-discharge options that allow a mother to leave within 12 to 24 hours of delivery. One reason for this change is that hospitals throughout the country are trying to cut down on skyrocketing health care costs. Shorter stays also reflect a changing view of the new mother as someone who is not ill, although she still requires time to recover and build up her strength.

In the first weeks after delivery, the mother's body undergoes dramatic changes—inside as well as out. The uterus, stretched bigger than a watermelon, shrinks to the size of a large grapefruit. This process, called *involution,* can cause cramps or afterpains that range from mild to severe for up to two weeks, particularly in women who have had other children. This discomfort peaks in the first two or three days after delivery and feels sharpest during breast-feeding because nursing releases a chemical called oxytocin that intensifies the contractions.

The body sheds the by-products of pregnancy in *lochia,* a vaginal discharge that may contain clots as big as quarters and initially is bright red. Lochia turns pinkish brown after two or three days, then creamy or yellow, and continues for four to eight weeks after delivery.

RECOVERY

It takes a while for the mother's body to return to normal. She usually loses about 11 pounds at birth and an additional four to five pounds in the following weeks. Four to eight weeks are required for the reproductive organs to return to normal. From the two-and-a-half pounds it weighs at delivery, the uterus must shrink back to a few ounces.

If the mother does not nurse, menstruation resumes in about four to 10 weeks. Breast-feeding delays menstruation because prolactin, the hormone involved in milk production, suppresses the hormones needed to trigger ovulation.

A mother's body will provide clues if something is amiss in her recovery. Among the warning signals new mothers should watch for are the following:

- A temperature of 100 degrees or higher, which, after the first 24 hours, could indicate infection.

- Changes in the lochia—foul smell, large clots, return to bright red bleeding, excessive amount—that might be caused by retained fragments of the placenta, by infection, or by overexertion.

- Tenderness or redness of the breast, which could be the result of a clogged milk duct (massage may relieve it) or infection.

- Pain or tenderness in the calf, possibly caused by a blood clot.

- Urgency of, frequency of, or burning during urination, signals of a urinary tract infection.

POSTPARTUM DEPRESSION

For the mother, the high of delivery may lead to an emotional low, known as postpartum depression. This time of fatigue, anxiety, and fluctuating moods is so common that obstetrics texts list it as a normal consequence of delivery. For most women, the condition is fleeting. For others, the depression, combined with fatigue and the new demands of the newborn, can persist for weeks and even months. In any case, pregnancy and childbirth are major life events for every woman and everything about and within her changes. Time is needed to achieve a new sense of balance and to adjust to the demands a new baby brings.

Fathers, too, may suffer postpartum blues. If they were actively involved in childbirth preparation and in the delivery, they may feel left out afterward, when the full impact of having another family member hits them for the first time. Just like new mothers, they must adjust to the often unsettling realities of life with a newborn.

Recently, scientists began to explore the possibility that there also exists a condition that goes beyond postpartum depression. This condition, known as postpartum psychosis, results in overwhelming depression and, often, in violence on the part of the mother. Little is known at this time, however, about this particular condition, and some scientists feel that it may not actually occur as a result of a birth.

BREAST-FEEDING

At one time most middle- and upper-class women bottle-fed their babies. Today, an increasing number of mothers, as well as the medical profession, believe breast milk is better for the child. Breast-fed babies have fewer illnesses and a much lower hospitalization rate, and their

A woman breast-feeds her baby. Many women today favor this method over bottle-feeding because it provides a variety of health benefits and may even enable the mother to pass her immunities on to her child.

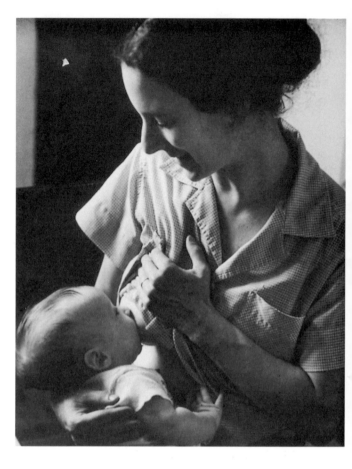

mortality rate is lower as well. Breast milk seems not only to prevent or lessen disease but also to help bring infection under control. When breast-fed babies do fall ill, they recover more quickly. Some scientists argue that breast milk passes on the mother's immunities to the baby. Breastfed infants are also less likely to become obese or develop allergies. Benefits of breast-feeding can also be psychological, as the process of nursing may reinforce the bond between mother and child.

There are valid reasons for a mother to choose not to breastfeed and to use a bottle occasionally or exclusively. According to the American Council on Science and Health, at least 20% of women are unable to breast-feed after their first deliveries; 50% of new mothers encounter significant difficulties in nursing. Women with inverted, or turned-in, nipples or those with very large breasts may encounter special difficulties in trying to nurse. Sometimes the woman's breasts become inflamed, or she must take medications that would be dangerous for her infant. Other times the infant is unable to suckle vigorously enough to get an adequate milk supply. Likewise, babies who are fed with bottles during an extended stay in the nursery or intensive care unit may not "take" the breast afterward.

Whatever the pros and cons, bottle-fed babies grow up just as healthy and happy as breast-fed ones. Infants do not live on milk alone; love and security are far more significant.

THE FIRST MONTH

Some people refer to the month after birth as the "fourth trimester." It certainly is a time of change and development for the new arrival— and for his or her parents.

Early Development

A baby's lungs begin working in the fluid-filled womb, practicing for the moment when it will swallow its first breath of air. While passing through the birth canal, the baby's chest is compressed, and some of the fluid in its lungs is squeezed out. With the first breath, the tiny sacs, or alveoli, within the lungs begin to open, pushing out the rest of the fluid. The lungs expand with each successive breath, as more air sacs open. Most babies can clear the fluid from their lungs on their own. Sometimes the birth attendant will suction mucous and fluid from the baby's mouth and throat to allow for easier breathing.

Newborns take about 30 to 50 breaths each minute and always inhale through the nose (which is why it is so important to keep that organ clear). Some babies do not establish a regular breathing pattern immediately, however, and skip breaths periodically, particularly when in active sleep or while sucking or crying. This usually is not dangerous in a healthy infant. But if the baby is at risk, the intensive care nursery staff will monitor its breathing to make sure the baby is taking at least 30 breaths a minute.

Because the lungs do not function before birth, a special circulatory system bypasses the lungs, diverting most of the blood to the heart and brain. Small amounts of blood enter the vessels of the lung, but the fluid in the lung creates resistance, which pushes the blood back through the ductus arteriosus, a small opening into the heart.

The very first breath, along with other complex changes in the blood's oxygen supply, decreases the resistance within the lungs and enables blood to enter. The ductus arteriosus thickens; within about three weeks it closes completely. If it remains open—a condition known as patent ductus arteriosus—the baby will not receive an adequate oxygen supply and will appear blue. Surgery may be necessary to close the ductus.

Shortly after the first cry, the newborn's heart rate speeds up to 175 to 180 beats per minute. After four to six hours it slows to 115 beats per minute. At 12 to 24 hours it rises again and then levels off at about 120 beats per minute. The range of normal heart rates in healthy newborns is from 100 beats per minute while sleeping to 120 to 150 beats per minute while awake. Blood pressure is also highest immediately after birth and descends within several hours.

The baby's liver faces an important task after birth: the breakdown of bilirubin, an orange or yellowish pigment found in bile. In the month before birth, the mother's liver breaks the bilirubin down. As the baby's liver takes over the process, the baby may appear yellowish, or jaundiced. This condition occurs in about half of full-term babies and 80% of all preemies. As has been mentioned, in some cases, phototherapy—exposure to bright light to accelerate bilirubin breakdown—is necessary.

At birth an infant can digest simple carbohydrates, proteins, and fats. Gradually more enzymes are produced to aid in the breakdown of foods. The salivary glands are immature; saliva is usually not produced for about three months. The baby's stomach empties intermittently, starting within a few minutes of a feeding; its control of the muscles in the stomach is immature, so some feedings may be spit up, or regurgitated.

Full-term babies have their first bowel movements within 12 to 48 hours after birth. Usually the stools consist of meconium, a thick, tarry, dark green waste material formed before birth. Subsequent bowel movements tend to be green or yellow and liquidy if the baby is breast-feeding and paler in color if the baby is on formula. Some babies have several bowel movements a day others have one every two or three days.

Most newborns begin urinating at birth or shortly thereafter. Normal urine in early infancy is straw-colored and almost odorless. Mothers

SUDDEN INFANT DEATH SYNDROME (SIDS)

S IDS, or crib death, is the most common cause of death for infants less than a year old. Each year about 7,000 babies succumb to this mysterious illness. Premature and very small babies are the most vulnerable.

In most cases, a seemingly healthy infant, usually one to seven months old, is put to bed according to the daily routine established by the parents. The baby may have a slight cold or cough but nothing that would alarm his or her parents. When the parents return to the crib, however, they find that the child is dead.

With SIDS there is no sign of a struggle, nor does the baby suffocate in the blankets. Autopsies generally reveal, at most, a minor degree of inflammation of the upper respiratory tract or signs of infectious disease. Consequently, it is often impossible to determine the cause of death.

Physicians know of no way to predict or prevent crib death. In fact, they know more about what does not cause SIDS than what does: It is *not* triggered by external suffocation, vomiting, choking, contagious disease, bottle-feeding, or hereditary predisposition.

There are some precautions parents can take. Highly sensitive electronic monitors can be set up to alert them if their child stops breathing during sleep. Monitoring is recommended if a baby has had a "near-miss" episode, that is, if on an earlier occasion he or she had stopped breathing but was discovered and resuscitated in time to prevent death.

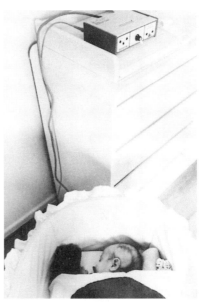

An infant's sleep is monitored by an instrument that measures breathing patterns. These devices are often used to alert parents in cases where there is reason to suspect that SIDS may occur.

may notice blood on the diapers of baby girls. This "pseudomenstruation," or false menstrual bleeding, is the result of the withdrawal of the mother's sex hormones from the baby's body.

During their first month of life, babies tend to curl up, regardless of the position they are laid down in. The main reason for this is that their heads are very large in relation to the rest of their bodies, and their neck muscles are too weak to support the heavy head. In all babies, muscle control begins at the top and gradually moves downward. By the end of the fourth week, a baby can lift its head for at least a few moments. A newborn's brain is about one-quarter the size of an adult's.

Babies, like most adults, spend their first month in one of two states: They are either completely asleep or awake and alert. For a baby, sleep consists of deep, or quiet, sleep and rapid-eye movement, or active sleep (the type associated with dreaming in adults). Newborns have no sense of day or night. They sleep as much as they need to—sometimes up to 16 hours a day. Infants often drift into sleep randomly throughout a 24-hour period, even while sucking on a breast or

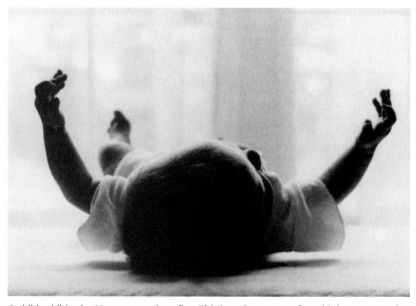

A child exhibits the Moro, or startle, reflex. This impulse, present from birth, causes an infant to throw out its arms and legs if it is alarmed or handled roughly.

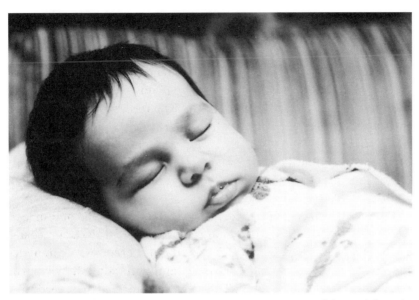

Newborns sleep as many as 16 hours a day. They have no concept of day or night and take several months to develop sleeping patterns that mirror their parents'.

a bottle. It takes several months for them to "learn" a sleeping-waking schedule.

Pediatricians break down the alert stage into four different categories: drowsy or semidozing, wide awake, active awake, and crying. Crying serves many purposes. It may distract the baby from hunger and pain (and alert the caregiver to these problems), and it may help the baby discharge energy.

Babies are born with certain built-in reflexes that they lose and relearn months later. If placed on their stomachs, they flex their arms and legs as if they are about to crawl (known as the prone-crawl reflex). They grip their fingers tightly around anything placed in their hands (referred to as the grasp reflex). If held up on a firm surface, they will take steps, as if they were walking. If startled or handled roughly, they throw out their arms and legs, instinctively seeking support (known as the Tap Moro reflex).

All of a baby's senses operate from the moment of birth, but each infant has to learn how to process the information the senses provide. Newborns can see, but they are extremely nearsighted and focus only

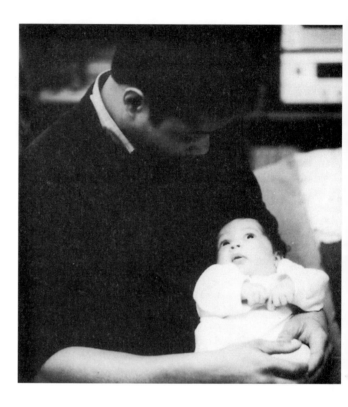

A newborn gazes at her father. Even very young babies are fascinated by faces and quickly learn to identify their parents or other primary caregivers.

on objects about eight to 10 inches from their face. Researchers have found that even at the earliest stages, babies like to look at faces and will look at a face longer than at any other object or picture.

Long before birth, babies can hear sounds made outside the womb. Loud noises startle newborns, but recordings of a heartbeat—the sound a fetus lives with inside the womb—may soothe them. By the end of their first month, infants can recognize the voices of those who matter most in their life. Although they may not understand words, they respond quickly to the speaker's tone, crying when they hear shouting or calming down when their mother or father croons softly to them.

Babies are born with built-in "tastes." Given something bitter, acidic, or sour, they turn away or cry. Offered some slightly sweetened water, they suck longer and harder. They also respond to touch. When stroked on the cheek, they will turn their head in that direction. They seem to like warm, soft pressure and motion, whether they are "riding" in a parent's arms, a stroller, or a car seat.

During their first month, babies live from moment to moment. They forget immediately about objects they can not see. They do not reach for something bright and shining, but they may kick with pleasure when such an object appears within their limited range of vision.

THE NEW FAMILY

The first month after a baby's birth is a time of transition for the family. The parents have gone through a major life event and may feel overwhelmed by the changes the baby has brought. They need time to

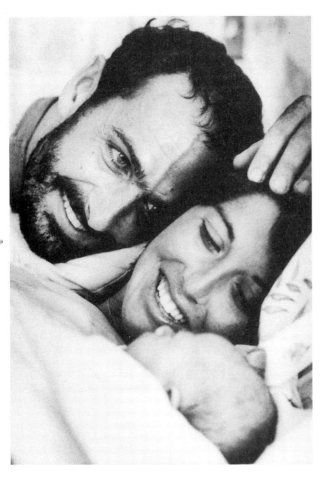

The months before and after the birth of a child are a time of transition. Most parents agree that this physically and emotionally challenging period is also profoundly rewarding.

adjust and to make room in their lives for the newest member of their family. The new arrivals also need time to take their unique place within the family and to begin their lifelong exploration of the world they have just entered.

APPENDIX

FOR MORE INFORMATION

The following organizations can provide more information about pregnancy, birth, and related issues.

Adoption

Division of Family and Youth Services
Department of Health and
   Social Services
350 Main St. 4th Fl.
P.O. Box 110630
Juneau, AK 99811-0630
(907) 465-3170
www.state.AK.US

Family Planning

Planned Parenthood Federation
   of America
810 Seventh Ave.
New York, NY 10019
(212) 541-7800
www.ppfa.org

Association of Maternal and Child
   Health Program
1220 19th St. NW, Ste. 801
Washington, D.C. 20036
(202) 775-0436
www.amchpl.org

Infertility and Childbirth

American Academy of Husband-
   Coached Childbirth
The Bradley Method
P.O. Box 5224
Sherman Oaks, CA 91413
(800) 423-2397 Pregnancy Hotline
   (except California, Hawaii, and Alaska)
(818) 788-6662

The American Society for
   Reproductive Medicine
1209 Montgomery Hwy
Birmingham, AL 35216-2809
(205) 978-5000
www.asrm.org

Nurse-Midwives

American College of
   Nurse Midwives
1522 K St. NW
Washington, DC 20005
(202) 347-5445
www.midwife.org

Teen Pregnancy

Children's Hospital of Los Angeles
4650 Sunset Blvd.
Los Angeles, CA 90027
(323) 660-2450
www.chla.usc.edu or www.chla.org

Adolescent Clinic
University of Colorado Medical Center
4200 E. Ninth Ave.
Denver, CO 80220
(303) 270-6659
www.uchsc.edu

Adolescent Clinic
New York Hospital-Cornell
   Medical Center
525 E. 68th St.
New York, NY 10021
(212) 434-5500
www.med.cornell.edu

Adolescent Clinic
Hospital for Sick Children
555 University Ave.
Toronto, Ontario M5G 1X8
Canada
(416) 813-1500
www.sickkids.on.ca

APPENDIX

FURTHER READING

American College of Obstetricians and Gynecologists. *Exercise during pregnancy and the postpartum period.* Technical Bulletin, vol. 189, 1994.

American Medical Women's Association. *Guide to Pregnancy and Childbirth.* New York: Dell, 1996.

Asimov, Isaac. *The Human Body: Its Structure and Operation.* New York: New American Library, 1963.

Bode, Janet. *Kids Having Kids.* New York: Watts, 1980.

Creasy, Robert, and Dianne Hales. *New Hope for Normal and Problem Pregnancies.* New York: Berkley, 1984.

Eisenberg, Arlene, Sandree Eisenberg Hathaway, and Heidi Eisenberg Murkoff. *What to Expect When You're Expecting.* New York: Workman, 1992.

Friedman, Rochelle and Bonnie Gradstein. *Surviving Pregnancy Loss: A Complete Sourcebook for Women and Their Families.* Secaucus, NJ: Citadel, 1996.

Gabbe, Steven, Jennifer Niebyl, and Joe Leigh Simpson. *Obstetrics: Normal and Problem Pregnancies.* New York: Churchill Livingstone, 1986.

Kitzinger, Sheila. *The Complete Book of Pregnancy and Childbirth.* New York: Knopf, 1980.

Leach, Penelope. *Your Baby and Child.* New York: Knopf, 1985.

Miller, Jonathan. *The Facts of Life.* New York: Viking, 1984.

Olds, Sally, Patricia Ladewig, and Marcia London. *Maternal Newborn Nursing: A Family Centered Approach.* 5th ed. Menlo Park, CA: Addison-Wesley, 1998.

Pasquariello, Patrick S. *The Children's Hospital of Philadelphia Book of Pregnancy and Child Care.* New York: Wiley, 1999.

Pool, Catherine M. and Elizabeth A. Parr. *Choosing a Nurse-Midwife: Your Guide to Safe, Sensitive Care During Pregnancy and the Birth of Your Child.* New York: Wiley, 1994.

Richards, Arlene Kramer, and Irene Willis. *What To Do if Someone You Know Is Under 18 and Pregnant.* New York: Lothrop, Lee, and Shepard, 1983.

Romero, Roberto, et al. *Prenatal Diagnosis of Congenital Anomalies.* Norwalk, CT: Appleton & Lange, 1988.

Rushnell, Elaine Evans. *My Mom's Having a Baby.* New York: Putnam, 1980.

Smith, Anthony. *The Body.* New York: Viking Penguin, 1978.

Tapley, Donald F., and W. Duane Todd, eds. *The Columbia University College of Physicians and Surgeons Guide to Pregnancy.* New York: Crown, 1988.

Wilson, Christine Coleman, and Wendy Roe Hovey. *Cesarean Childbirth.* New York: Dolphin, 1980.

Wilson, Joseleen. *The Prepregnancy Planner.* New York: Doubleday, 1986.

APPENDIX

GLOSSARY

Abortion: The termination of a pregnancy; may occur naturally as a miscarriage or be induced artificially, especially by a doctor.

AIDS: Acquired immune deficiency syndrome; an acquired defect in the immune system, thought to be caused by a virus (HIV) and spread by blood or sexual contact or through nutritive fluids passed from a mother to a fetus; leaves people vulnerable to certain, often fatal, infections and cancers.

Alpha-fetoprotein: Protein manufactured in the liver of a fetus and by adults with certain pathological conditions; in fetuses, abnormally high or low levels, which can be detected by amniocentesis, may indicate certain birth defects or increased risk of pregnancy complications.

Amniocentesis: A test for genetic defects in an unborn child; chromosomes in fetal cells drawn from fluid inside the amnion are examined for abnormality; cannot be performed until the mother is 14 to 16 weeks into a pregnancy.

Amnion: One of the membranes surrounding a fetus during development.

Apgar: A numerical score that determines an infant's physical condition based on the infant's heart rate, respiration, muscle tone, response to stimuli, and color one minute after birth.

Braxton Hicks contractions: Irregular tightening of the muscles of the uterus that occurs late in pregnancy.

Breech birth: A common abnormality of delivery wherein the infant's buttocks, rather than head, appear first; in this case, doctors often perform cesarean sections in order to prevent any complications

Cesarean section: Delivery of a baby through an incision in the mother's uterus and lower abdomen.

Chorion: One of the membranes surrounding the fetus in early stages of development; later it helps to form the placenta.

Chorionic villi sampling: Method of testing for genetic defects very early in a pregnancy (8 to 10 weeks); the chromosomes in cells taken from the chorion are examined for abnormality.

Cocaine: A topical anesthetic applied to mucous membranes that, when used for nonmedical purposes, can produce a psychological dependence classified as drug abuse.

Congenital: Acquired during development rather than through heredity.

Dilation: Expansion of an orifice, especially of the cervix to ten centimeters to allow a baby to pass through during delivery.

Down's syndrome: A variety of congenital mental retardation, ranging from moderate to severe, caused by the presence of an extra chromosome; marked by certain physical abnormalities.

Eclampsia: A convulsive disorder occurring between the 20th week of pregnancy and the end of the first week postpartum, often preceded by pre-eclampsia and characterized by high blood pressure during pregnancy; it can jeopardize the life of a mother and her baby if left untreated.

Ectopic pregnancy: A pregnancy in which a fertilized egg implants itself in the fallopian tube, abdominal cavity, ovary, or cervix instead of in the uterine cavity.

Embryo: The developing fertilized egg during the first eight weeks after conception.

Episiotomy: An incision made to enlarge the vaginal opening to allow the baby to pass through during birth.

Fetal alcohol syndrome: A cluster of physical and mental birth defects resulting from a mother's chronic alcoholism during pregnancy.

Fetus: The developing embryo during the period beginning in the ninth week after conception

Herpes virus: A family of viruses that contain large amounts of DNA; they include herpes simplex, which causes painful sores on the mouth (simplex I) or on the anus and genitals (simplex II); the latter simplex can be passed on to a fetus.

Implantation: Process whereby a blastocyte (an embryonic cell) imbeds itself in the lining of the uterus six or seven days after fertilization.

Infertility: Physical inability to produce offspring; in women an inability to conceive; in men an inability to fertilize eggs.

Involution: The shrinkage of the uterus that occurs in the first weeks after delivery.

Lanugo: Fine downy hairs that cover a fetus and remain evident on a premature baby.

Linea nigra: The dark line that forms down the center of the mother's abdomen during pregnancy.

Lochia: The discharge of by-products from the uterus after delivery.

Marijuana: Plant that, when ingested or smoked, produces a feeling of euphoria; certain forms are being used experimentally to alleviate symptoms of severe glaucoma.

Miscarriage: The expulsion of an embryo or fetus, usually between the third month and viability.

Neural tube defects: Congenital malformations of the brain, spine, or abdominal wall caused by failure of the neural tube to close in development.

Ovulation: Release of an egg cell, or ovum, from the ovaries; the time at which a woman is most likely to become pregnant.

Oxytocin: Hormone that triggers uterine contractions; also signals mammary glands to stimulate the release of milk.

PUBS: Percutaneous umbilical blood sampling; a prenatal diagnostic test in which a needle is inserted directly into a baby's umbilical cord to obtain a blood sample for testing.

Placenta: The organ that develops during pregnancy to supply the fetus with oxygen, food, water, and nutrients from the mother's bloodstream and to carry waste back to the mother's body for disposal.

Rh factor: A chemical substance found in the red blood cells of some people (i.e., they are Rh-positive); if red blood cells from an Rh-negative fetus enter the bloodstream of an Rh-negative mother, they may trigger destructive antibodies that can endanger future pregnancies with Rh-positive fetuses.

Rubella: German measles, an acute infectious disease that can cause birth defects if the mother contracts it during pregnancy.

Tay-Sachs disease: An inherited disease most prevalent in Jewish children of eastern European descent.

Toxemia: Blood poisoning that spreads the products of a locally focused bacteria throughout the body, thus producing general bodily symptoms.

Ultrasound: High-frequency sound waves used in a diagnostic test to perceive and recreate images, especially of fetuses.

Vernix caseosa: A protective coating that forms over a fetus.

APPENDIX

INDEX

APPENDIX

PICTURE CREDITS

Diane Hales is the author of *The Family* in Chelsea House's Encyclopedia of Health. She is the author or coauthor of nine books, including *Case Histories* in Chelsea House's Encyclopedia of Psychoactive Drugs, *An Invitation to Health: Your Personal Responsibility, The U.S. Army Total Fitness Program, The Comptete Book of Sleep,* and *New Hope for Problem Pregnancies.* She is a contributing editor of *American Health* magazine and a frequent contributor to other magazines, including *McCall's, Redbook,* and *Parade.* Ms. Hales has also written for the *Washington Post,* the *New York Times, American Medical News, Medical World News,* and *Psychiatric News.*

C. Everett Koop, M.D., Sc.D., currently serves as chairman of the board of his own website, www.drkoop.com, and is the Elizabeth DeCamp McInerny professor at Dartmouth College, from which he graduated in 1937. Dr. Koop received his doctor of medicine degree from Cornell Medical College in 1941 and his doctor of science degree from the University of Pennsylvania in 1947. A pediatric surgeon of international reputation, he was previously surgeon in chief of Children's Hospital of Philadelphia and professor of pediatric surgery and pediatrics at the University of Pennsylvania. A former U.S. Surgeon General, Dr. Koop was also the director of the Office of International Health. He has served as surgery editor of the *Journal of Clinical Pediatrics* and editor in chief of the *Journal of Pediatric Surgery.* In his more than 60 years of experience in health care, government, and industry, Dr. Koop has received numerous awards and honors, including 35 honorary degrees.